Once a Month

An Open Letter from a PMS Sufferer...

It is difficult for me to put into words how much I love and admire Katharina Dalton, and how important I consider her books to be on both a personal and a professional level.

Dr. Dalton was the first physician to begin diagnosing, treating and researching premenstural syndrome—a problem that has diminished the lives and potential of women for thousands of years. In the face of controversy and considerable professional risk, she has moved premenstrual syndrome into the mainstream of accepted medical practice throughout most of the world. Her papers and medical texts have enabled physicians everywhere to help their own patients, and her lay text, *Once a Month*, has made it possible for women to identify their problem and seek the help they need.

Personally, I credit *Once a Month* and Dr. Katharina Dalton with saving my sanity and my life. By the time I found this book I was at the end of my rope. My undiagnosed illness was taking three weeks of each month and I was in the emergency room of Duke Hospital almost every month to relieve the pain and nausea associated with menstrual migraine. My doctor told me that he didn't know what was wrong, but that he believed I had a menstrually-connected illness that would probably abate with menopause. At the age of 27, I was being handed a 20-year sentence of pain and suffering for myself and those who loved me. I began to feel I had reached the point where I no longer wanted to live.

Then my mother read about the first PMS clinic in the United States, scheduled to open in Boston, treating PMS sufferers along lines laid down by Dr. Katharina Dalton. When *Once a Month* was handed to me in Boston, my first feeling was a flood of relief: just to know that I was not suffering alone! It gave me renewed hope for my life. I thought that any problem this well-documented and studied for over 30 years would be readily recognized and treated in the United States. Unfortunately, for most women in the U.S. in 1980, this was not true.

For this reason, a group of women suffering from PMS joined hands to see that Dr. Dalton's work could be made known to women in this country and that their illness would be respected and diagnosed. We founded the National PMS Society to help millions of women, each of whom thought she was suffering alone. For the last six years, the Society has been dedicated to establishing support groups and services for sufferers, and Dr. Katharina Dalton has been our constant source of inspiration and information.

In a way, *Once a Month* was the catalyst for a revolution in women's medical care in the United States. Today, we understand our illness and we are no longer willing to accept the "neurotic lady" treatment silently. We are no longer willing to listen to physicians who tell us that our pain and suffering is a part of being a woman that must be accepted, or that PMS is a psychological problem. We also know now that we are not alone. I will never understand how 27 million women were convinced that they suffered an illness unheard of or unexperienced by anyone else.

The woman with PMS today has to deal with a confusing barrage of "breakthrough" therapies, conflicting diet plans, over-the-counter medications, vitamin recommendations (some of which have proven dangerous), here-today gone-tomorrow clinics, and books. The only defense we have is to educate ourselves about our problem so that we can make informed decisions. I highly recommend that a woman begin this educational process by reading *Once a Month*, the original PMS handbook, first written in 1978 and now in its third revised edition. Dr. Dalton has never stopped researching and trying to improve her understanding of premenstrual syndrome. As she has increased her understanding, she has carefully and continuously updated *Once a Month*.

When trying to find a medical opinion I can trust, I am always reassured by Dr. Dalton's lack of selfish motives or commercial interests. She simply has a missionary zeal to help women who suffer as she once did.

Dr. Dalton and I both look forward to the day when this condition will attract the funds that are really needed to discover the cause and cure of premenstrual problems in all women. Until then, her work is the standard against which all others are measured. She is the godmother of modern health care for women; a brilliant, warm, honest physician. For her dedication to the improved health and happiness of all women, my husband thanks her, my children thank her, my family and friends thank her, and most of all... I thank her.

Lindsay Leckie
Founder, National Premenstrual Syndrome Society, Inc.

About the Author

Katharina Dalton was born in England, in 1916. Her early training was as a chiropodist at the London Foot Hospital, where she wrote *Essentials of Chiropody*, now a basic textbook. Widowed with one child during the war, she started medical training at the Royal Free Hospital, worked in the evenings, remarried and had three more children. In 1948, she qualified as an M.D. and entered general practice where, during the first two months, she identified and successfully treated six women suffering from pre-menstrually-related asthma, epilepsy and migraine. For 23 years she continued researching premenstrual syndrome in her general practice. This interest resulted in 1953 in the first paper in British medical literature on the premenstrual syndrome, written in collaboration with Dr. Raymond Greene. In 1954, her work with premenstrual syndrome patients at University College Hospital, London, led to her establishing there the world's first and oldest premenstrual syndrome clinic, which she still maintains and where, in conjunction with her Harley Street practice, she continues her studies into premenstrual syndrome and related illnesses.

Dr. Dalton is now an acknowledged authority on the part played by menstrual dysfunctions in confused and criminal behavior, accidents, drug abuse and morbidity. Her work on premenstrual syndrome and its treatment with progesterone therapy is applied in factories, schools, prisons, shops and hospitals, and she has received widespread recognition for her research. She has been awarded the Charles Oliver Hawthorne BMA prize for outstanding research in general practice on three occasions, and has also received the Upjohn Fellowship, the Charlotte Brown prize from the Royal Free Hospital, and the British Migraine Association prize from the Royal College of General Practioners, of which she was a founding member. In 1971 she became the first woman President of the General Practice section of the Royal Society of Medicine. In 1980 she was an expert witness in two cases of murder in which premenstrual syndrome was accepted as a factor causing diminished responsibility, thus making legal history in Britain. She was awarded the Fellowship of the Royal College of General Practioners in 1982.

Her books and publications have been translated into 12 languages, and include *The Premenstrual Syndrome* (1964), *The Menstrual Cycle* (1970), *The Premenstrual Syndrome and Progesterone Therapy* (1977, 2nd ed. 1984), and *Depression after Childbirth* (1980). She has lectured extensively to both medical and lay audiences all over the world, and has made numerous radio and TV appearances in Europe and the United States.

Dr. Dalton is married to a Unitarian minister and has four children and five grandchildren.

Dr. Katharina Dalton's

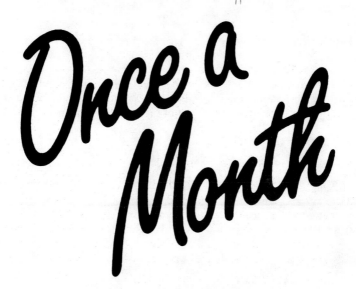

Once a Month

THE ORIGINAL PREMENSTRUAL SYNDROME HANDBOOK

Third Revised Edition

R. REGINALD
The Borgo Press
San Bernardino, California ▫ MCMXC

©1979, 1983, 1987 by Katharina Dalton

First published in Great Britain by Fontana Paperbacks 1978

First U.S. edition published in 1979, second (revised) U.S. edition published in 1983, third (revised) U.S. edition published in 1987 by
    Hunter House Inc., Publishers
    P.O. Box 1302
    Claremont, CA 91711
    U.S.A.

Grateful acknowledgement is given the following for permission to reprint copyrighted material:

"The Importance of Diagnosing Premenstrual Syndrome" from *Health Visitor*, 1982.
"Legal Implications of PMS" from *World Medicince*, 1982

Library of Congress Cataloging-in-Publication Data:

Dalton, Katharina, 1916-
    Once a Month

    Includes index.
    1. Premenstrual syndrome. 2. Menstruation disorders.
I. Title. [DNLM: 1. Premenstrual Syndrome—popular works.
WP 550 D149o]
RG165.D34   1987   618.1'72   86-7263
ISBN 0-89793-043-6

Cover design by Qalagraphia
Set in 11/12 Goudy Old Style by Richmond House
Printed and bound by Delta Lithograph Co., Valencia, CA
Manufactured in the U.S.A.

9 8 7 6 5 4 3 2   Third edition

1339 6524

Contents

Contents (Continued)

List of Figures

List of Figures (Continued)

Preface to the Third Edition

The need for a third edition is a clear indicator that the demand for authentic information on the premenstrual syndrome is in no way slowing down. Nor, regrettably, are the torrents of misinformation, false information, mythical treatments and armchair theories. Indeed, it is these outpourings that are creating the confusion, not merely among the unfortunate sufferers of premenstrual syndrome, but also among the public, social workers and other health professionals. This adds a greater urgency to the need to provide a third edition based on the experience accumulated during more than 38 years of continuous work with this pernicious disease.

There have been considerable advances in our knowledge of a woman's reproductive processes since this book was first written in 1977. These include the realisation that each woman's menstrual cycle follows her own individual pattern, which can vary considerably from woman to woman and yet remain normal; an appreciation that hormones are multifunctional; and an understanding of their behavior, their transport through the body and their interactions within the target cell. Of particular importance are the recognition of progesterone receptors in the midbrain and the value of an estimation of the binding capacity of sex hormone binding globulin (SHBG). But there is still much ignorance and many questions that need to be answered. New knowledge on the subject is eagerly awaited to help in solving some of the remaining mysteries.

Meanwhile, there remains a need for self-help groups to assist women in making the connection between their symptoms and menstruation; to instruct in menstrual charting; to teach the essential dietary rule of eating some starchy food every three hours; and to point the sufferer toward sympathetic medical practitioners ready to prescribe effective treatment to eliminate monthly problems. Groups can agitate for the inclusion of premenstrual syndrome in the medical curriculum at both undergraduate and postgraduate levels, ensure that adequate funds are available for research and clinical trials, and educate society to recognize that premenstrual syndrome is a hormonal and not a psychological disorder. In 1986, American women showed their strength by overturning the American Psychiatric Association's desire to see premenstrual syndrome labeled as a mental disease.

In this edition a new chapter, "Clearing the Confusion," has been added to help readers to verify the authenticity of what they read and hear about premenstrual syndrome. It also explains the difficulty of trying to diagnose premenstrual syndrome correctly, using conventional methods of diagnosis. There is new information in almost every chapter, although some are more altered than others.

"Nature knows no pause in progress and development and attaches her curse on all inaction." Both aspects of Goethe's nineteenth-century saying are to be found in the story of premenstrual syndrome. The ongoing progress and development is to be found in my many writings from 1953 to the present, and is reflected in the neverending stream of women referred daily for diagnosis and treatment. The other side, Nature's curse, is experienced by those countless women whose premenstrual sufferings continue because of the unwillingness of practitioners to use effective progesterone treatment until its success has been proven in double-blind placebo controlled trials. To some that may sound a reasonable excuse for inaction, but let us take a lesson from history. Scurvy was the major cause of mortality and morbidity among sailors on long sea voyages, until the sixteenth century when the Dutch discovered the value of a diet containing citrus fruits with which to combat scurvy. Nevertheless, it was not until 1932 that vitamin C (ascorbic acid) was identified as the curative agent in the fruit. In those earlier years no one felt the need to wait three centuries until science found the evidence — "the proof of the pudding lay in the eating," so to speak — and consequently many thousands of lives were saved from the ravages of scurvy. Today, the women suffering from premenstrual syndrome who have been properly treated with progesterone know how very effective it is. Do the others have to wait 300 years until we know the exact mechanism of its action, or are they deserving of treatment now?

During the preparation of this third edition that question has been in the forefront of my mind, alongside another one: how can I encourage my colleagues to learn the necessary new skills to enable them to correctly diagnose and properly treat premenstrual syndrome? This book has been written in the firm belief that all who read it with an open and unprejudiced mind will be able to learn a great deal about premenstrual syndrome and the reason for its treatment with progesterone. They will also appreciate that it is a very real disease which can have extremely serious consequences for some of its sufferers, but a disease that has responded magnificently to progesterone treatment ever since this was first used in 1948.

It now remains for me to continue with my work of healing and to express my gratitude to all those patients who have taught me so much; also to the many colleagues who have contributed to the development and increase of my understanding of endocrine involvement in the disease, particularly my daughter, Dr. Maureen Dalton. These thanks would not be complete without an acknowledgement of the invaluable contribution of my hardworking staff, especially Wendy Holton and Jane Rogers. As always, your thanks and mine must go to my husband, the Rev. Tom Dalton, for all his support and untiring determination to maintain a high standard of readability for your enlightenment and pleasure. Finally, my acknowledgement to William Heinemann Medical Books Ltd. for permission to reproduce Figures 7 and 8 from my book *Premenstrual Syndrome and Progesterone Therapy*.

Katharina Dalton
London, 1987

Preface to the Second Edition

In 1954, speaking to the General Practice Section of the Royal Society of Medicine, I ended my paper with the words:

> "The cost of progesterone therapy is high, but when this is weighed against the price in terms of human misery, suffering and injustice, it is seen as a justifiable expense opening up a new vista of Medicine."

That vista is still opening up and during the last few years considerable progress has been made in the appreciation and understanding of menstrual problems and their treatment by the caring professions and also by the general public.

At the symposium on Premenstrual Syndrome at the International Congress of Psychosomatic Obstetrics and Gynecology held in Berlin in September 1980, it was agreed that the premenstrual syndrome was a hormonal disease, therefore it was more suited for study by international meetings of endocrinologists rather than by psychologists. Of course there will always be those who disagree and suggest other approaches, which is as it should be, provided they are talking about the same diagnosed disease and have tried the same treatments, comparing them with other treatments to find the most successful.

New issues have emerged, such as the legal implications and the feminist movement. The premenstrual syndrome should not be a feminist issue. It is a hormonal disease, which deserves sympathy and understanding and requires to be diagnosed and treated.

This edition has been widely revised in the light of the findings of the past four years and includes a new Appendix on "Legal Implications." It is as up-to-date as it is possible to be, in the hope that the disease will be more commonly recognized, correctly diagnosed and properly treated.

Katharina Dalton
London, 1983.

Preface to the First Edition

This book is dedicated to the thousands of women who have confided in me the most personal and intimate details of their lives and from whom I have learned so much.

I am deeply grateful for the help received from all my family. To Drs. Maureen and Michael Dalton who have been my most severe critics; to Mrs. Anita Dalton and Mrs. Wendy Holton who have patiently typed, corrected and retyped the manuscript before it was ready for submission to the publishers; to my niece, Mrs. Sherryl Machray for the artwork; to Mrs. Sharlynn Orr who has kindly adapted my work for America; and most of all to my long-suffering husband, Rev. Tom Dalton for his invaluable ghost-writing of the entire book.

Finally, my acknowledgment to David Duff and Tandem Press for the excerpt from *Albert & Victoria*, and the Journal of the Royal College of General Practitioners for permission to reproduce Figure 11.

Katharina Dalton
1978

Introduction

Once-a-month, with monotonous regularity, chaos is inflicted on American homes as premenstrual tension and other menstrual problems recur time and time again with demoralizing repetition. This book explains how these premenstrual problems can be completely relieved with the proper treatment, just as the pains of childbirth are today universally treated with pain-relievers and anesthetics.

It has also been written to help men to understand the capricious and temperamental changes of women, so that the image of woman as uncertain, fickle, changeable, moody and hard to please may go, to be replaced with the recognition that all these features can be understood in terms of the ever-changing ebb and flow of her menstrual hormones.

It was as long ago as 1948 that I came across my first case of premenstrual asthma, which responded successfully to treatment with progesterone. Before a month had passed a further case of asthma, two of epilepsy and one of migraine had been found, all related to menstruation. However, for the premenstrual syndrome to be properly appreciated it must be recognized in all its full variety. Following a recent television documentary on the subject which showed only four presentations — an alcoholic, a baby batterer, a husband-beater and a neurotic — the hospital's postbag was filled with letters which suggested that the program had been an eye-opener to many viewers, whose letters contained such comments as:

"It was such a relief to know that so many other women experience the very real and deep feelings of anger, hatred and depression that I feel at period times."

"I'm just like that woman."

"I never told anyone because I thought they would never believe me."

It is hoped that this book will open many more eyes for it is estimated that there are in America today over 5½ million women with incapacitating monthly problems which can and should be eased.

The first step is to bring the subject out into the open, and not to sweep it under the carpet. Menstruation should be a subject that can be discussed as openly as sex; anywhere, by anybody, not merely in the bedroom or doctor's office. We still suffer from the utterly Victorian attitude in which heroines in novels never menstruate. If women themselves do not yet associate the changes in their body and psyche with the changes in menstrual hormones, how can one hope that men will be able to understand them? After all, men don't even experience it. There must be a general recognition of the physical and psychological changes in a woman which occur like a flash of lightning before menstruation, and which are not due to personality inadequacies.

While accepting that fatalities from the premenstrual syndrome or period pains are rare and the suffering is short-lived, ending with menstruation, nevertheless the suffering, unhappiness and social consequences of it are without limitation.

One gynecologist ranks the premenstrual syndrome as the commonest cause of marital breakdown. In a general practice survey in England, 75% of a sample of 521 women complained of at least one premenstrual symptom. In Britain, the attempted suicide rate shows that there is a seven-fold increase in the second half of the menstrual cycle compared with the pre-ovulatory half. Shoplifting is thirty times commoner in the second half of the cycle. Of 132 women who were currently under the care of the Premenstrual Syndrome Clinic at University College Hospital, London, during December 1977, 37% had a previous mental hospital admission; 34% had attempted suicide or homicide; 9% had alcoholic bouts; 6% were referred because of actual child abuse and a further 4% sought treatment because of a fear of their injuries to their children becoming public knowledge; 6% had a history of criminal behavior, such as smashing the windows of the Social Services headquarters, and assaulting police or neighbors; 7% had premenstrual epilepsy and 5% had premenstrual asthma.

These are no trivialities but are of vital concern to the patient, her family, society, and maybe even a nation. This is shown in the following extract from *Albert & Victoria*, David Duff's book on the married life of Queen Victoria (London: Muller, 1972):

"One of the reasons why Victoria continued to bear children was her belief that, by doing so, she kept her grip on Albert... When she was pregnant he was always kind, thoughtful, attentive of her every wish. Here was a problem that he could understand, a train of events to which he could attend. But he knew nothing of the imponderable in women. He was completely inexperienced. He did not appreciate the unreasoned emotions which surged like a maelstrom in Victoria's brain. Albert's answer to all the problems of life was to exercise reason... When Victoria began throwing things and screaming her accusations into his face, he would retire to write a paper on the cause of the outburst. She would then receive a letter beginning "Dear Child" and containing simple ingredients for an antidote to emotion. This did not help matters. Albert soon learned that any action that he took at such times was wrong. Answering back led to faster, louder vituperation. Remaining quiet was classified as insulting. Retiring behind a locked door eventually led to an attack upon its panels by royal fists... Even (Lord) Melbourne, a past master at dealing with women, had on one occasion quavered and feared to sit down as the fire blazed in the eyes of the eighteen-year-old queen. A cabinet minister was known to fly from her presence, too frightened to follow the rule of withdrawal. Thus Albert looked forward to the period of pregnancy — it gave emotion a reason."

The premenstrual syndrome knows no geographical, social, racial or economic boundaries; its sufferings and tragedies are

spread evenly throughout our society. For many it is sufficient reassurance to know that other normal women also
experience the same monthly feelings, while the knowledge
that there is a satisfactory answer provides them with hope
for the future.

1

The Curse of Eve

Once a month women are reminded that their reproductive system is still in the process of evolution. But it is no good waiting another two or three million years for Mother Nature to iron out the flaws. In the short term it is better to try to understand the way our body works, the problems with which the silent majority tries to cope, and how best they can be helped.

The other natural functions of the body, such as growth, respiration, digestion, and excretion go on day by day without pain. Indeed, if pain is present it is abnormal, a cause for concern, and a thorough search is made to find and eradicate the disease. On the other hand, the two natural feminine physiological processes, menstruation and childbirth, are seldom completely without pain. It is thought that less than one woman in five goes through her childbearing years without at some time suffering from period pain or premenstrual tension. It is now universally accepted (although it was not always so) that women experiencing pain during labor are deserving of relief with analgesics and anesthetics, and they even go into training for this one-day event with weekly relaxation classes. One hopes that the time of enlightenment is not too far off when treatment for the relief of period pains and premenstrual problems will be accepted as the natural right of every woman the world over.

Menstruation represents a failed pregnancy, and only occurs if the woman is neither pregnant nor breastfeeding. It was therefore a comparative rarity in primitive society. A normal woman could expect to menstruate once a month for an average of 35 years, but our great-grandmothers, who breastfed their families of twelve children as the only known method

1

of contraception, averaged 11 years of intermittent menstruation. By contrast, today's mother of two, who breastfeeds for an average of three months, may expect almost continuous menstrual cycles for 33 years.

Anne, 34 years, was brought to the doctor's office by her Catholic priest because of a severe asthma attack which accompanied her last menstruation. She was asked if asthma had also accompanied the menstruation before her last one. She took a few minutes to think about it before admitting "I was only eighteen at the time and I can't really remember." She had fourteen children, and for the last 16 years had either been pregnant or breastfeeding.

Pain is not the only symptom associated with menstruation: there are also the psychological and bodily symptoms which come out of the blue once a month, usually just before menstruation, and come under the omnibus heading of the Premenstrual Syndrome. Examples include Barbara and Carol.

Barbara wrote:

I have such drastic changes in personality before a period I think I am going mad. I cannot understand how I can feel so differently towards my children, one day loving and caring for them and the next day being so hateful and rough, so bad-tempered and smacking them for nothing. How guilty I feel when I see my own daughter, aged five, copying me and smacking her dolls."

Carol wrote:

"I have one fantastic week each month, but after ovulation my whole body changes, my breasts start to swell, I look five months pregnant with a swollen tummy, my chest is tight and I just can't breathe because of asthma. There is usually a migraine on the first day of menstruation."

Relief is possible for women with painful periods and also for those with premenstrual symptoms, like Barbara and Carol.

However, first it is necessary for them to realize the association between their symptoms and menstruation, which means either the patient herself must recognize it, or her husband, mother, close friend, or doctor has to. Once the problem is recognized, treatment is available, as will be seen in later chapters.

It has been said, "Man is born to suffer, but woman is born to suffer more," and sometimes it seems that no efforts are being made to ease woman's sufferings. Consider this list of excuses culled from recent letters:

"It's not fatal and doesn't last long"

"She'll get over it"

"Cool it, lady, you're neurotic"

"Things will be easier when you're married" . . . "or have had children" . . . "or when the children have grown up"

"Learn to live with it and take more exercise"

"Accept the symptoms — you're not going mad — and learn to relax"

"Only because you've not enough to do" (to a woman with three children, all under school age)

"You're working too hard" (one child at school)

"You're only trying to jump on the bandwagon like 90% of other women"

And so the excuses go on, with the adoption of an ostrich-like attitude to once-a-month problems, and with no efforts made to solve them.

There is nothing new about these menstrual problems. Even Hippocrates, the father of medicine, blamed premenstrual tension on "the agitated blood of a woman seeking a way of escape from the womb." Primitive man found it difficult to understand how women could lose blood every month, yet neither be ill nor die. Even today many men are amazed that women can accept the regular loss of blood so cheerfully, when they themselves panic each time they have a nosebleed or cut a finger. But it is only rarely that women complain of the blood itself; it is how they feel and look, and the pains they suffer, that worry them. When primitive tribes lived in isolation there might be only one menstruating woman present at any one time. It was natural then to endow her with supernatural powers, normally ascribed to gods. These powers included an ability to stop hailstorms, whirlwinds, and lightning if she went out into the open unclothed. Menstrual blood was also thought to be endowed with valuable properties, such as the power to extinguish fires, temper metals and fashion swords as well as to protect men against wounds in battle. A thread soaked in menstrual blood was considered a valuable treatment for epilepsy and headache (today we often find that once menstruation starts, the premenstrual epilepsy or headache is relieved).

Myths about menstruation are worldwide. In some parts of the world the presence of a menstruating woman was believed to cause harm, being able to sour wines, blight crops, rust iron or bronze and turn copper green. She could cause cattle to abort, seeds to dry up, fruit on trees to die, bright mirrors to become dulled, the edge to be taken off sharpened metal, a hive of bees to perish, the strings of harps to break, clocks to stop, and linen to turn black. Can one wonder that women in India went into *purdah* at these times?

During the Middle Ages it was believed that menstruation demonstrated the essential sinfulness and inferiority of women, who were therefore forbidden to attend church or take communion, a custom still observed in the Greek Orthodox Church today. For this reason also, Orthodox Jewish women are instructed to make themselves plain and unattractive during menstruation to avoid exciting their husbands sexually. Following menstruation, the woman is required to undergo a ritualistic cleansing by immersing herself three times in a "body of water."

In different countries there are many local customs associated with menstruation, which are concerned chiefly with the local industries and fear of their failure. In Indonesia, menstruating women may not enter tobacco fields or work in rice paddies. In Saigon they may not be employed in opium factories, lest the opium turn bitter. In France and Germany they were excluded from the wineries and breweries lest they turned wine or beer sour; and in the Canary Islands today women are not allowed in the grape-crushing area. In France, the presence of a menstruating woman during the boiling process in sugar refineries might turn the sugar black. Parsee women in India may not look at a fire lest their glance extinguish it. In Syria, if pickling is done by menstruating women it is believed the food will be putrefied. In South Africa, menstruating women may not come into contact with cattle for fear their milk will turn sour. Until the last century in England it was believed that if menstruating women salted meat it would not keep.

The problems associated with menstruation are obviously not new; they represent the eternal mystery of women. What is new is the changing attitude of the medical profession which now contains a few doctors, far too few, who have interested themselves in these problems and have shown that they can be successfully treated, and treated without witchcraft. Other doctors are trying to learn how to correctly diagnose and properly treat these problems, but are often confused by the bewildering amount of misinformation and, far too often, wrong information that is constantly being presented to them by people with little or no practical experience of premenstrual syndrome. These doctors see this shamefully neglected subject of menstruation, with its complexity of symptoms which can change a woman from Jekyll to Hyde within minutes, as a challenge to be met.

THE MENSTRUAL CYCLE

To ensure the continuation of the human species, nature has evolved, in a woman, a system which produces an egg cell at precisely the right time for it to be fertilized by the sperm of the male. Research has shown that this is not the simple process we used to believe it was, it is really very complex. There is no need for us to go into all the details, however; nature's basic system is the menstrual cycle, which can be explained in quite simple terms and still be a correct account of the process of childbearing.

Woman is born with two ovaries containing thousands of immature egg cells. Each month, in response to a message from the pituitary gland, one of the unripe egg cells develops inside a tiny microscopic ring of cells, which gradually increases to form a little balloon or cyst called the Graafian follicle. These cells of the ovary make the menstrual hormone, *estrogen*, about which we will be hearing much more later. When the little egg cell is fully developed it appears as a blister on the surface of the ovary, and under a further message from the pituitary gland it bursts and releases the mature egg cell. When this occurs it is known as *ovulation*. The egg cell makes its way down the Fallopian tubes to the womb, a journey that takes about fourteen days. Meanwhile, the yellow scar tissue left behind when the blister bursts fills up with new cells which produce the second important menstrual hormone, *progesterone*. The progesterone acts on the lining of the womb to turn it into a soft spongy layer in which the fertilized egg cell can embed itself if a pregnancy occurs. During intercourse, millions of male sperm are projected into the vagina, and journey through the womb up into one of the Fallopian tubes in an attempt to fertilize the egg cell so that conception will occur and pregnancy can begin. The fertilized egg passes into the womb and becomes embedded in the new soft lining, where it develops into a baby. Following successful fertilization, progesterone will continue to be produced to protect the developing baby from being rejected by the mother's womb.

However, if the egg cell has not been fertilized, the production of progesterone begins to fall. About 14 days after ovulation the soft spongy lining of the womb, which is then not needed, disintegrates and is shed, together with the unfertilized egg cell. This is *menstruation*, which represents a failed pregnancy.

NORMAL VARIATIONS OF MENSTRUATION

Each woman's menstrual cycle is unique and individually her own, consequently there are considerable variations. The menstrual flow, which is the disintegrated lining of of the womb, may appear as a pink watery discharge, or as thick red blood, or be reddish-brown or black, and it may contain shreds or small blood clots. All these variations are normal and healthy. Similarly, menstruation may occur every 21 or every 36 days, or anywhere in between, and it will still be considered as normal and compatible with full reproductive functioning. A variation in the length of a woman's cycle of up to four days month by month is also normal and almost to be expected. Ovulation occurs no earlier than 14 days before menstruation so, taking into account the different lengths of menstrual cycles, ovulation can occur as early as day 10 or as late as day 22.

There are also variations in the amount of menstrual flow on different days of menstruation. Some women have the heaviest flow on the first, second, and third day and then stop abruptly. Others have moderate loss for a day or two and then the heaviest loss on the third or fourth day. Then there are those women who have a scanty loss for a day or two with the flow gradually increasing in amount. It is important for the doctor to know which is the day of heaviest loss because, in premenstrual syndrome, the spontaneous relief of symptoms will not occur until the day of heaviest loss. So, for some women, symptoms may well occur during the early days of menstruation.

PHASES OF THE MENSTRUAL CYCLE

The menstrual cycles of different women vary considerably in length, but for the purpose of understanding the hormonal changes during the menstrual cycle it is convenient to divide it up into seven phases of four days each, which assumes the woman has a precise cycle of 28 days. It will be noticed that in the seven phases there are no two phases which have the same levels of hormones circulating in the blood. (Figure 1)

The phases are:

Days   1–4   *Menstruation*, with rising estrogen levels

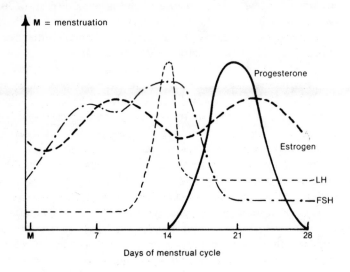

Figure 1 Menstrual hormone variations during the menstrual cycle

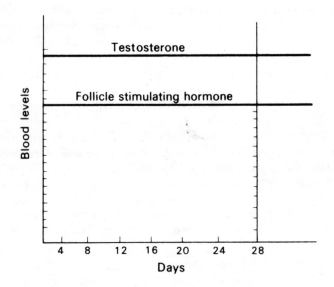

Figure 2 Male hormone levels during a month

Days   5–8   *Postmenstruum*, with peak estrogen levels

Days   9–12   *Late postmenstruum*, with falling estrogen levels

Days   13–16   *Ovulation*, with low estrogen and peak levels of follicle stimulating hormones and luteinising hormones

Days   17–20   *Post-ovulation*, with rising estrogen and progesterone levels

Days   21–24   *Early premenstruum*, with peak estrogen and progesterone levels

Days   25–28   *Premenstruum*, with falling levels of estrogen and progesterone

For comparison, the steady daily levels of male hormones are shown in Figure 2.

The first four days of menstruation and the last four days before menstruation are known as the *paramenstruum*. It is a useful term and is used in surveys, for these days occur regardless of the length of a woman's cycle. Any adjustment due to a cycle length longer or shorter than 28 days is made in the late postmenstruum. In long cycles the postmenstruum will be longer than eight days, while short cycles will have a short postmenstruum. Readers should note that the progesterone which is present from ovulation till menstruation is a natural hormone, and should not be confused with the man-made progestogens or progestins, which have completely different actions. (See also pp 185–186)

The attitudes of women to regular menstruation vary considerably. Some think of it as a sign of normality and an indication of good health. Others regard it as a sign of femininity with maternal attributes, or an assurance that, though they are not pregnant now, they are fertile. Menopausal women see menstruation as a sign of their youthfulness to which they are so anxious to cling, while those who see menstruation as a once-a-month nuisance, to be tolerated as Mother Nature's wish, wonder why medical scientists have not given more thought to the abolition of the associated ailments and complaints.

A study of the words used throughout the world to describe menstruation is fascinating. In Jamaica, Nigeria, Egypt and Mexico, words are used to imply a state of ill-health or pain, such as "being unwell" or "having the blues." In Yugoslavia, Mexico, Egypt and the Philippines, the menstrual bleeding is often personified as a "visitor," while in Britain it may be "the curse," or given the familiarity of an old friend like "Charlie" or "Archie." In Nigeria and Jamaica, young girls are taught about "growing up" using the analogy of "flowers and bees," so that when menstruation occurs it is called "flowers." Women in Egypt and Korea often use terms associated with sanitary pads and bathing. In Indonesia the words used are associated with pollution or with purification. In the Philippines the phrase "desire for abortion" is sometimes used when describing menstruation.

Psychologists object to the use of the word "curse," claiming that it conditions women to expect trouble with menstruation. On the other hand, women have as many menstrual problems in Nigeria and Jamaica, where the word "flowers" is used. There is no doubt that psychological factors do play a part in menstrual problems, but this is only secondary to the hormonal effects.

2

Mood Swings

"Tell me Doctor, why does my wonderful wife, with her perfect figure and lovely nature, suddenly spit with rage for no obvious reason once a month?"

There are innumerable answers to that question. Most likely the blame will be laid on external events, while the upset of chemicals which occurs within her body at the time of menstruation will be overlooked. These chemical changes can produce changes in personality or sudden swings of mood as menstruation approaches, followed by a return to normality as soon as or shortly after the menstrual flow starts. This is known as the premenstrual syndrome (or, more familiarly, as PMS). Doctors use the word "syndrome" for a group of complaints or symptoms which cluster together.

The mood swings may vary from being a minor nuisance to becoming a major catastrophe. There may just be an unexpected reaction to a trivial irritation, a hilarious conversation abruptly ended by a cutting remark or a blunt rebuke, or a loss of a sense of humor. On the other end of the scale there may be violent verbal abuse or smashing and throwing of things. At the far extreme lies the possibility of suicide, homicide, or infanticide. It is easy for an observer to attribute this to a lack of self-control, or call it a temperamental outburst, or even evidence of the woman's true character. Too rarely are these mood swings properly attributed to the natural ebb and flow of the menstrual hormones, over which the woman has such little control.

These premenstrual mood swings are widespread and occur in at least half of all women. This means that there is also another 50% of women who do not experience them at all, and do not know what the other half are suffering. Why this fortunate 50% do not suffer is explained in Chapter 16. Men do not experience such changes in hormone levels. The male sex hormones, or chemical messengers, remain on an even keel day by day throughout the month, as shown by the levels of follicle stimulating hormone (FSH) and testosterone in Figure 2. How different are the levels of the woman's four sex hormones, *follicle stimulating hormone (FSH), luteinising hormone (LH), estrogen* and *progesterone*, which vary day by day throughout the month, as shown in Figure 1. Only a slight imbalance in any of these levels is enough to cause problems for a woman.

The term "Premenstrual Syndrome" is used to embrace *any symptoms or complaints which regularly come just before or during early menstruation, but are absent at other times of the cycle.* It is a precise definition, and means that the symptoms must be present each and every month. Symptoms must occur premenstrually, and there must be a symptom-free phase each cycle. It is the absence of symptoms after menstruation which is so important in this definition.

There is an endless list of different symptoms which may occur in this syndrome, including tension, depression, tiredness, irritability, backache, asthma, sinusitis, epilepsy, and weight-gain. Fortunately, no woman suffers from all the possible symptoms. All these individual symptoms can also be experienced by men, but in the male they are random complaints, not occurring once every month. It is only in women that we find these symptoms regularly related to menstruation.

Premenstrual syndrome needs to be differentiated from *menstrual distress.* Menstrual distress covers *symptoms present throughout the menstrual cycle with increased intensity before or during menstruation.* Such symptoms may be intermittent, as with headaches, or continuously present throughout the day, as with anxiety or depression.

Most sufferers of the premenstrual syndrome suffer from more than one symptom at the same time. For instance, many sufferers will notice weight-gain and an increase in tension before the onset of a premenstrual headache. The removal of only one symptom, for example by giving a tranquilizer to ease the tension, will be of little help to the gain in weight and the headache.

It is also important to remember that the definition of the premenstrual syndrome requires not only the presence of symptoms related to menstruation, but also the complete absence of these symptoms at other times of the menstrual cycle. It is this absence of symptoms, and the change of mood after menstruation back to being a happy, energetic, vivacious woman once more, which clinches the diagnosis.

This letter from a patient illustrates the point:

> "I have suffered from the usual premenstrual symptoms for five years and my tension, irritability and depression were put down to nerves, but I must say I could never understand this as it was only at certain times of the month that I seem to be so nervous, tense and depressed and lacking confidence. I found that about ten to twelve days before my period I felt as if something was draining out of me, and as if something chemical was happening, and so often I tried to pull myself together at this time and it just never worked. I get so irritable and nervous a week before that I just want to shut myself up in a house; I feel as if I can't go out to work and socially I avoid any sort of engagement at this time of the month. At other times I'm O.K."

The exact type and severity of symptoms varies with each individual, but in every sufferer her own time-schedule of discomfort is the same, month by month, or rather, cycle by cycle. The easiest tool for recognizing the relationship of symptoms to menstruation, and the absence of symptoms at other times of the cycle, is the simple menstrual chart shown in Figure 3 and discussed fully in Chapter 3.

The start of the mood swings may be quite sudden and the victim may surprise even herself by her own outrageous behavior. It has been described as "a blanket of fog which enfolds me," while a 20-year-old student thought of it as "changing from top gear to bottom in the car." In other cases, the beginning may be quite gradual, symptoms becoming worse day by day. Problems may start at ovulation and last the full fourteen days until menstruation, so that one sufferer felt she had been "crazy for half my life," or they may occur only days or hours before the onset of menstruation. Even if they only last for a few days, they can still be a great source of concern, as one letter-writer described:

> "Every month it is the same, and the thought of being knocked out for a couple of days each month for the next twenty or so years fills me with a sense of desperation, as it is such a waste of days which could be used for living instead of for wallowing in."

Indeed, in premenstrual epilepsy the attack may be measured in minutes or hours rather than in days. The symptoms tend to last longer as one approaches the menopause. A 42-year-old teacher wondered if "this gradual lengthening of the negative mood would mean that there may soon be a time when there is no bright spell left at all." It was good to be able to reassure her that, however long the premenstrual mood lasted, there would always be a bright spell once a month after menstruation, for premenstrual symptoms do not start earlier than fourteen days before menstruation, however long or short the menstrual cycle may be.

For many women the onset of menstruation works like a charm, and as the blood flows the relief has been likened to "a cloud lifting," or "the curtain opens again." The very occasional sufferer may even be freed from her symptoms a day or just a few hours before menstruation starts. Yet others may find relief is slower, and they may not regain their joy of living until a couple of days after menstruation has finished. When it's over, one may hear a loving husband announce "She's now like the woman I married!"

Age and pregnancy are two factors which tend to make the symptoms of the premenstrual syndrome become worse and last longer, so it may be first diagnosed in the thirties. In fact, in 1963, Dr. T. Stacy Lloyd of Virginia suggested the name "Mid-Thirty Syndrome" for this same collection of symptoms related to menstruation. By the mid-thirties women have been married, been on the pill and stopped; they have had their pregnancies and possibly been sterilized; all of these being factors which increase the incidence and severity of premenstrual syndrome. It was noted at the International Symposium on Premenstrual Syndrome held in South Carolina in 1983 that many speakers, when introducing their papers on different aspects of their work, described the age of the patients they had studied, and these were invariably in the mid-thirties. They described women who had attended Premenstrual Syndrome Clinics and had been diagnosed as suffering from the disease. But all too often it is the young adolescents and those in their early twenties who suffer in silence without being diagnosed; instead, they are thought to be bad-tempered, miserable and lazy; they are unloved, and so end up in bad company, leading to yet more problems. The title "Mid-Thirty Syndrome" fortunately never caught on, and one hopes it will be forgotten as it is unfair to those in other age groups.

This increase in severity is more marked in the years just before menopause, so much so that all too often the premenstrual mood swings are blamed on menopause. A woman of fifty years exclaimed "I've been in menopause for the last fifteen years — when will it ever end?" It is more likely that she had been suffering from undiagnosed premenstrual syndrome for all that time.

Fortunately, there is an end to this exclusively feminine syndrome, in that when the menopausal changes are complete, menstruation ends and so do the monthly fluctuations of mood and other symptoms. Menopause marks the end of childbearing. Ovulation ceases, and gradually women's hormones readjust, and then progesterone is no longer required. This is the time when one may look forward to an era of serenity.

3

Clearing the Confusion

Without a doubt there is much confusion about premenstrual syndrome. The medical profession is confounded by it, no matter whether they are gynecologists, psychiatrists or endocrinologists; even general practitioners, who see the condition first and are in an ideal situation for treating it, are equally perplexed. Few consultants know anything about it, even though premenstrual syndrome invades every specialty. Add to this the appalling ignorance and utter befuddlement of the media's presentations on this subject, and it is only too easy to understand how the bewilderment continues to grow. It is hoped that this chapter will help to clear away these mists of confusion.

In such a situation it is essential to establish a definition of the disease in question. The definition of premenstrual syndrome, as already indicated in Chapter 2, is "the presence of any symptoms or complaints which regularly come just before or during early menstruaton but are absent at other times of the cycle." The precise definition means that three requirements must be fulfilled for a correct diagnosis:

1) Symptoms must be present every month for at least the previous three months.

2) Symptoms must be present premenstrually, and cannot start before ovulation.

3) There must be complete absence of symptoms after menstruation for a minimum of seven days.

The successful treatment of any disease depends on the accuracy of the diagnosis. To achieve that accuracy, a doctor must take into consideration symptoms, signs and investigations. That means the doctor listens to the patient's account of the complaint; takes note of any signs of disease which may be revealed by examination; and studies the results of blood tests, X-rays and other investigations. The doctor accepts the patient's account of her symptoms (be they a sore throat or a pain in some part of the body), and having examined for signs and considered the results of tests, he makes his diagnosis and treats appropriately. All too often, when women come to their doctor claiming they have premenstrual symptoms, the doctor accepts their claim at face value without appreciating the need to further check the diagnosis before giving treatment.

TIME RELATIONSHIP OF SYMPTOMS TO MENSTRUATION

With premenstrual syndrome the doctor must verify the diagnosis, for in premenstrual syndrome there are no special symptoms indicative of the disease; all the symptoms can be complained of by men, children and postmenopausal women. The disease only affects women of childbearing age. There are no specific signs discovered on examination, and no definitive investigations. How, then, can an accurate diagnosis be made in a disease which has no special symptoms, no specific signs, and no distinctive investigations? The one clear diagnostic clue is the time relationship of symptoms to menstruation. It therefore becomes necessary to find a new method of diagnosis which will enable this crucial time relationship to be clearly established.

Psychiatrists frequently use questionnaires as part of their diagnostic procedures, asking the patient numerous questions and analyzing the replies. This is a useful method in psychiatry, enabling numerical scores to be obtained for an individual's level of, for example, depression, anxiety, neuroticism, or marital stability. This score can then be used to compare the results of different treatments.

MENSTRUAL DISTRESS QUESTIONNAIRES

In 1968, Rudolph Moos designed the Moos Menstrual Distress Questionnaire, which proved most effective in demonstrating the amount of distress caused by menstruation. The questionnaire has been used in some tests for premenstrual syndrome, but it cannot differentiate premenstrual syndrome from menstrual pain or distress. In the test, a woman is asked to complete 47 different questions each night on a six point scale. These includes questions such as "Today did you have any orderliness? ... excitement? ... loneliness?" It is a method which relies on the honesty, reliability and determination of the candidate. While it is easy to complete the questionnaire and carefully consider your reply for one — or even seven — consecutive days, one doubts the accuracy of the method when, as in Sampson's tests in 1978, women completed the questionnaire every single day for six months. There is always a need for caution in interpreting the results of questionnaires when they are used for purposes other than those for which they were designed.

The information obtained on such questionnaires needs to be prospective, obtained daily, rather than retrospective, obtained by such questions as "During the days before menstruation do you suffer from ... ?" Today, women have been educated by the media to know that headaches, bloatedness, backache and irritability tend to occur premenstrually, so if they suffer from such symptoms at all they may automatically assume that their headache or other symptom occured before menstruation.

THE MENSTRUAL CHART

If one is to rely on the help of the patient in making the diagnosis, it is important to keep the diagnostic aids simple, in order to eliminate the possibility of inaccuracy and guesswork. The menstrual chart shown in Figure 3 is widely used by doctors, and it is easy enough for anyone to copy out for themselves. The purpose of the chart is to provide the precise information necessary to make an accurate diagnosis of premenstrual syndrome by recording the actual dates of men-

Name _____ Year _____

	Jan.	Feb.	Mar.	Apr.	May	Jun.	Jul.	Aug.	Sep.	Oct.	Nov.	Dec.
1												
2												
3												
4												
5												
6												
7												
8												
9												
10												
11												
12												
13												
14												
15												
16												
17												
18												
19												
20												
21												
22												
23												
24												
25												
26												
27												
28												
29												
30												
31												

Figure 3   Menstrual chart

struation and the days when symptoms or complaints are present. The woman is asked to choose only her most important symptoms, those complaints she would most like to lose. These symptoms are then given symbols, such as "H" for headache, "X" for quarrels, "T" for tension. A small letter, "h," "x," or "t," can be used for mild symptoms, and the capital letter for symptoms that are really severe. There is never a need to use more than one letter for any one symptom. The letter "M" may be used to represent menstruation, although some use "P" for period (it doesn't matter what symbols are used). The chart is completed each night with a record of whether the symptom was present or absent, and whether it was severe during that day. Some women like to insert a dot on those days when they feel well; this ensures that they complete the record. It should be completed daily regardless of the phase of the menstrual cycle or the apparent cause of the symptom. Doctors interpreting the chart are fully aware that there may be other circumstances which cause the same symptoms. For instance, spending a few hours watching your son having his lacerated leg sutured in an emergency room may well cause you to feel tense, irritable or depressed, regardless of the phase of the cycle. Again, you may well feel exhausted or have a headache after an all-night delayed flight returning from a holiday.

From using a menstrual chart it becomes immediately obvious whether symptoms are clustered around menstruation, as in Figure 4, or occur haphazardly throughout the month, as in Figure 5. It is easy to see the duration of menstruation or of symptoms, and to notice if the menstrual cycle is short, for the "M"s will be going up the chart, or if it is long, for the "M"s will be going down the chart. Furthermore, it is not necessary for the woman to be menstruating to obtain information as to the cyclical character of her symptoms. Cyclical symptoms can occur at times of occasional missed menstruation or even before menstruation has begun, at the menopause, or after the removal of the womb or ovaries.

One mother, a sales executive who was herself receiving treatment for premenstrual syndrome, was disturbed to find that her well-behaved daughter of thirteen had occasional "off" days when she would be rude and lazy, which was out

Jan. Feb. Mar. Apr.

	Jan.	Feb.	Mar.	Apr.
1				
2				
3				
4				
5				
6				
7				
8				X
9				X
10		X		X
11		X		M·X
12		X	X	M·X
13		X	X	M
14		X	M·X	M
15		X	M	M
16	X·B	M·X	M	M
17	X	M	M	
18	X	M		
19	M·X			
20	M			
21	M			
22	M			
23				
24				
25				
26				
27				
28				
29				
30				
31				
Total				

May Jun. Jul. Aug.

	May	Jun.	Jul.	Aug.
1		M		
2		M		
3				
4				
5				
6				
7				
8			H	
9			H	
10			H	
11			H	
12			H	
13			M·H	
14			M·H	
15			M·H	
16			M	
17			H	M
18			H	M
19			M·H	M
20			M·H	
21			M·H	
22			M	
23		H	M	
24		M·H	M	
25		M·H	M	
26	H	M·H		
27	H	M		
28	H	M		
29	M·H	M·H		
30	M	M		
31	M			

Sep. Oct. Nov. Dec.

	Sep.	Oct.	Nov.	Dec.
1				
2				
3	B			
4	B			
5	B			
6	B			
7	B			
8	M·B			
9	M·B			
10	M	B		
11		B		
12		B		
13	M·B			
14	M			
15	M	B		
16	M	B		
17	M	B	B	
18		B	B	
19		M·B	B	
20		M	B	
21		M	B	
22		M	B	
23		M	M·B	
24			M·B	
25			M	
26			M	

M = Menstruation H = Headache

X = Tension B = Backache

Figure 4 Menstrual charts diagnostic of premenstrual syndrome

of character for her. Then the mother received reports from school that her daughter had occasional rebellious days during which she found it hard to accept discipline but easy to be rude. The mother carefully recorded the dates of these outbursts (shown on the chart in Figure 6), which occurred at intervals of 32–36 days. When later the daughter started to menstruate, the timing of her menstrual cycle averaged 35 days. In fact, this mother had diagnosed the premenstrual syndrome before menstruation had started. It is not necessary for ovulation to occur before the premenstrual syndrome develops.

Occasionally, the diagnosis may be made because the observations of others reveal the cyclical character of the symptoms. For instance, a legal executive took note of the days

	Jan.	Feb.	Mar.	Apr.		May	Jun.	Jul.	Aug.
1	X		X	M					H
2			X	M					
3			X	M		H	H		
4									
5				X					H
6				X		H		H	
7			M			H			
8	X		M·X				H		
9	X		M				H		
10		X	M				H		
11									H
12		M				M		H	
13		M	X	X		M			
14		M				M·H	H		
15		X				M		M	
16	X					M		M	
17	M					M		M	M
18	M					M	M	M	M
19	M	X				M	M	M	M
20		X		X			M	M	M
21			X				M	M	M
22			X			H	M		M
23	X					H	M		
24	X						M·H		
25	X								
26		X							
27				X					
28		X		M		H			H
29				M			H		
30	X			M				H	
31						H			
Total									

M = Menstruation   X =   Quarrels

H = Headaches

Figure 5   Menstrual chart with unrelated symptoms

when her secretary's typing deteriorated and she became aggressive, and when these revealed a pattern of recurring every 30 to 33 days, the boss advised her secretary to seek medical help. The value of similar information received from police, prison officers and medical records is mentioned in Chapter 14.

The PMT-Cator is a sophisticated circular diagnostic chart developed by the PMT Clinic, Dulwich Hospital, London, and is useful as a screening tool in a busy clinic. The woman chooses her five main symptoms to record daily, starting on

	Jan.	Feb.	Mar.	Apr.	May	Jun.
1					X	
2						X
3						X
4						
5						X
6						
7						
8						
9						
10						
11						
12						
13						
14						
15						
16	X					
17	X	X				
18	X	X				
19						
20		X				
21	X	X				
22						
23		X				
24			X			
25			X			
26				X		
27			X	X		
28				X		
29			X	X		
30			X			
31					X	
Total						

13 years old   X = rude or lazy

Figure 6 Chart of adolescent girl with cyclical symptoms before the start of menstruation

the first day of menstruation and scoring each symptom from 0 (none) to 3 (severe). There is a top disc designed to cover up previous recordings so that each night's entry will be unbiased.

At the end of the cycle the woman can remove the top disc and add up her score for the first seven days after menstruation, and her score for the last seven days before menstruation. If the final score for the premenstrual week exceeds 25, or if the premenstrual score subtracted from the postmenstrual score exceeds 14, a probable diagnosis exists. A definitive diagnosis of premenstrual syndrome cannot be made from a single disc, however; many women have severe symptoms for only three or four days in the premenstruum, and the presence of postmenstrual symptoms needs further investigation.

HORMONE BLOOD TESTS

Tests to determine the blood level of progesterone are of little value in the diagnosis of premenstrual syndrome, for low levels are also found in women who are not ovulating, although they do not necessarily suffer from premenstrual syndrome. However, recently a blood test that estimates the level of the sex hormone binding globulin (SHBG) binding capacity has proved valuable in premenstrual syndrome. My daughter, Dr. Maureen Dalton, showed in 1981 that 50 women suffering from severe, well-diagnosed premenstrual syndrome all had SHBG-binding levels below the normal level of 50–80 nmol/1 DHT, as compared with 50 healthy women who were adamant they did not suffer any premenstrual symptoms. (Figure 7) Furthermore, her work showed that SHBG levels rise when progesterone is administered, and the greater the dose of progesterone the higher the SHBG level. (Figure 8) Later work showed that if progestogens were administered, the SHBG levels were lowered. There are, however, limitations on this test's usefulness, for the woman whose blood is to be tested must be free from all medication (which includes analgesics, oral contraceptives, laxatives and vitamin preparations), must not be unduly obese or excessively hairy, and should not suffer from liver or

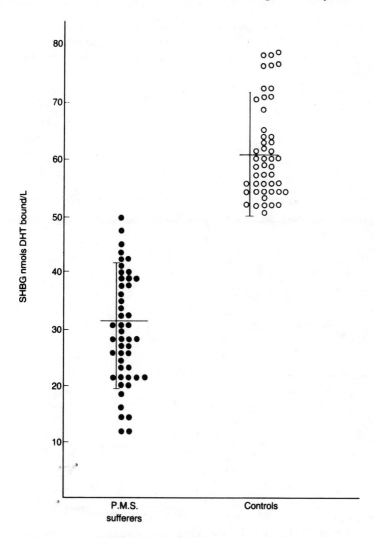

Figure 7 SHBG-binding capacity in 50 patients with
severe premenstrual syndrome compared with
50 symptom-free controls

thyroid disease. Furthermore, the blood must be centrifuged
and stored frozen until analyzed by the purified two-tier
method, which is at present only available at a few specialized
testing centers.

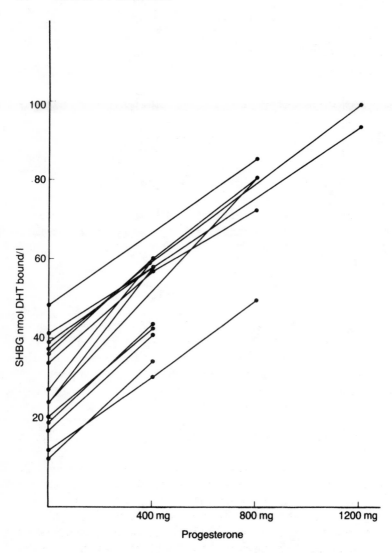

Figure 8 Effect of progesterone on SHBG levels

DIAGNOSTIC POINTERS

The menstrual chart requires a minimum of two months for completion and, as already mentioned, the SHBG test is not universally available; but there are occasions when one is anxious to make a rough diagnosis earlier. This can be done by considering those characteristics that are common to most women with premenstrual syndrome, usually referred to as "diagnostic pointers."

Medical students are taught that the onset of premenstrual syndrome is linked with PPPA: puberty, pregnancy, the pill, and amenorrhea, or absence of menstruation, such as occurs after anorexia nervosa or after serious illnesses or accidents. In the young adolescent it may result in an unexpected change of personality. One mother wrote:

> "For three weeks of the month our daughter is charming, capable and intelligent, then for the few days before her period she is sharp-tongued, impossible to live with, and seems to be boiling with rage."

Spasmodic dysmenorrhea, or severe colicky spasms of pain which start with the onset of menstruation, is unusual in sufferers of premenstrual syndrome (see Chapter 8). Because menstruation is practically painless and a non-event, many women with premenstrual syndrome initially fail to make the connection of their other symptoms with menstruation.

When, during pregnancy, menstruation stops and the blood level of progesterone rises to some 30–50 times the peak level reached during the premenstruum, women with premenstrual syndrome lose their symptoms. Many a husband has exclaimed, "I wish my wife could be forever pregnant."

The premenstrual syndrome may develop unexpectedly when menstruation returns after a pregnancy. If a pregnancy has been complicated by high blood pressure, swelling of the ankles, or an abnormally large gain in weight (signs of preeclamptic toxemia), or if it has been followed by puerperal or post-natal depression, then the chances are high, ten to one, that the unpleasant premenstrual syndrome will follow in its wake. What is worse, the premenstrual syndrome is likely to increase in severity after each pregnancy, even if the later pregnancies are normal.

The premenstrual syndrome may start when the woman is on the pill, or during the week when she is off it, but complaints are likely to be more marked and the bright and dull days more accentuated when pill-taking ends. Then the woman resumes her normal menstrual cycle, which may well be three or five weeks and not the precise 28 days ordained by the makers of the pill. Marriage is often given as another time at which the premenstrual syndrome started, but in these cases it may be that the observant husband has noticed mood swings and other symptoms, and related them to menstruation, while the woman had not noticed the relationship before. Again, pill-taking may have coincided with marriage.

It is often an outside observer who notices the mood swings first, usually the husband or mother, but occasionally an employer, social worker, friend or daughter. Following a television feature called *Pull Yourself Together, Woman,* a husband wrote:

> "I was so startled to recognize in all these cases the symptoms from which my wife has been suffering for the past eight years. The connection with the menstrual cycle may seem less direct but nevertheless the symptoms are heightened in the premenstrual period and are free thereafter. Briefly, they include acute anxiety and depression (in any order, as it seems impossible to distinguish cause and effect) manifested by physical symptoms of pressure on the head (variously described as an iron band around the head or a heavy weight at the back of the head) and dizziness; and by psychological symptoms such as agoraphobia, panic, guilt, obsessions and depressions, sometimes to the extent of suicidal notions."

Recently it has been recognized that premenstrual syndrome often increases in intensity following tubal ligation. Radwanska, Hammond and Berger of Illinois University showed that after women had the simple operation to block their fallopian tubes they subsequently produced less progesterone from their ovaries.

During adult life, sufferers tend to have large weight swings exceeding 28 lbs., although swings of 50 lbs. or more are not unusual. The lowest weight since leaving school is subtracted from the highest non-pregnant weight to measure the weight swing. It is irrelevant whether the individual is obese or slim at the time of interview.

Sufferers have difficulty in going long intervals without food, especially in the premenstruum, and may notice that they get faint, excessively tired, panicky or irritable. They also tend to suffer from uncontrollable premenstrual food cravings and binges, especially when they have deliberately refrained from food for a long time or when they have been dieting. This tendency is not due to a personality failure but is the result of the hormonal imbalance. It even occurs in baboons in the jungle, who go up into trees and, in isolation, gorge on unlimited amounts of honey during their premenstruum.

The tolerance to alcohol also varies during the cycle. Premenstrual syndrome sufferers usually find they can enjoy their favorite drink with no ill effects at other times, but in the premenstruum, even a reduced amount causes intoxication.

If the woman gives many positive answers to the diagnostic pointers listed above, there is every likelihood that in two months she will return with a positive chart. There are occasions when it may be worth giving a patient a therapeutic trial with progesterone before waiting for definitive diagnosis, but both the doctor and the patient should be aware that a positive diagnosis has not been made and, of course, she cannot be a candidate for any clinical tests.

An analysis was made of the final diagnosis in over 200 women who attended a premenstrual clinic. Its conclusions were that, while the menstrual chart is the only reliable diagnostic method for premenstrual syndrome, the SHBG estimation was more specific, more sensitive, and had a greater predictive value than the checklist score of diagnostic pointers.

4

Premenstrual Tension

Tension may be described in many ways, but the tension which occurs in the premenstrual syndrome has three parts to it: depression, tiredness and irritability. These three aspects are always present in premenstrual tension, although one of them may be more obvious than the others, if only temporarily so. Dr. Billig, in 1952, aptly described the depression as "the world looks like a sour apple," the tiredness as a "fall in energy," and the irritability as feeling "crabby"; and there are plenty of women who know exactly what he means.

These three symptoms may be interwoven, with each one creating equal stress, as *Dorothy's* letter shows:

"Premenstrual tension has been present throughout my reproductive life. I have seen my doctor many times but he has really been unable to help. Perhaps predictably, the condition has grown steadily worse in the years just before the marriage break-up, and much, much worse since. The strain is very great and well-nigh unbearable during the premenstrual time. I do not batter my children physically, but I do verbally, and I think that that can be almost as damaging, although I do try to explain to them why I behave as I do and apologize for it. The trouble begins as early as twelve to fourteen days after the beginning of the last period: the first sign is a disturbance of sleep. I get violent dreams and often wake, and when it is time to get up feel as though I have had no rest at all. The other half of the cycle I sleep perfectly soundly. Then I become so tense I positively shake and am so nervous and irritable that I am sorry for anyone who has to live with me. Quite often my heart starts to pound for no obvious reasons, as I have not been running or indulging in any violent exercise. I feel listless and apathetic, and often fall asleep during the day; on the other hand, the other half of the month I am energetic, hard working and clear headed. The onset of the period releases the tension but triggers off headaches which fluctuate from day to day for a couple of days. I cry at the drop of a hat during all this period, and find it hard to deal with any of the many problems objectively. Although I have been very depressed, I have never been put out of action, thanks probably to the good professional help. Apart from this misery I am healthy and active and very rarely ill."

Premenstrual tension, popularly abbreviated as "PMT," is only one aspect of premenstrual syndrome, which includes bodily or somatic symptoms as well as the psychological ones.

The tension may come on quite suddenly, with an inability to relax and feeling generally uptight. One housewife complained that when she was in this state she seemed to tremble so much that she even had difficulty threading a needle. Frequently, women are shy of mentioning premenstrual tension to their doctor, thinking that it is a common and minor complaint. Instead they seek what is known by the medical profession as a "passport symptom," or a somatic symptom like a headache, backache or 'flu, which they consider is more acceptable. One mother wrote:

"When I go to the doctor I am always conscious that I am not physically ill and so perhaps do not want to tell him all my, to other people, petty feelings. After all, one does not want to admit being a failure as a wife and mother."

Sometimes the tension reaches almost manic proportions, with such agitation and restless energy that the woman cannot calm down; she keeps walking up and down, or won't stop talking, and just repeats herself endlessly.

One husband was upset because:

"It's no use trying to tell her to relax, she just keeps

repeating herself and won't stop talking. New thoughts keep tumbling out. She accuses me of all sorts of things. She just goes on and on and on."

Premenstrual tension, like all other symptoms of the premenstrual syndrome, is always aggravated by other stress. None of us can totally free ourselves from the stresses of daily life, such as when extra work is demanded of us because co-workers are absent, or a strike occurs which hampers our normal activities, or when friends or neighbors are involved in a car crash or other accident. The usual effect of any of these stresses will be to cause an increase in the premenstrual tension when the time of the next menstruation approaches. On the other hand, good news will tend to ease the tension, and a winning bet or lottery ticket can be most beneficial in relieving premenstrual tension, but only for a month or two.

DEPRESSION

The depression may be so mild that the actual word is not used or is even denied. For example, the woman may say that she is fed up or down in the dumps, that she can't laugh easily and has difficulty in smiling, or that the whole world is against her but nobody cares. On the other hand, premenstrual depression may range to the other extreme, with the ever-present possibility of suicide, a risk which should be fully appreciated.

One husband wrote describing his wife's depression:

"I feel her life is at risk; she dreads these times so much it colors her whole life. She feels there is no hope."

A mother described her 20-year-old daughter's depression:

"These occurrences are so regular that for years I have associated them with periods. But when she approaches her doctor, usually in a state of panic, she is either told to go away and pull herself together, or is given tranquilizers, and on at least three occasions she has taken the lot and has had to have her stomach pumped out. When she is in this state she often proves violent and smashes things or hits her boyfriend. She also swallows vast quantities of alcohol and then sometimes cuts her wrists, always in the wrong direction. When she is herself after a period she is such a nice, kind and good-natured person."

A Washington, D.C., secretary ended her full description of premenstrual depression with the statement:

"The sad thing is that although suicidal thoughts cross my mind at this time, I am a very happy person ordinarily."

The MacKinnons, a husband and wife team of doctors, showed as long ago as 1956 that successful suicides predominated during the premenstruum. Studies of attempted suicides in hospitals in London and Delhi, and among the Samaritans in Los Angeles, have all confirmed that half of all women's attempts at suicide are made during the four days immediately before or the first four days of menstruation.

Although women make more attempts at suicide than men, the men succeed more frequently, though this masculine success rate gradually disappears after the age of 50 years. Dr. John Pollitt, speaking at the Royal Society of Medicine in 1976, suggested that:

". . . perhaps one reason for the female's lack of success is that the majority of attempts are made during the pre menstrual phase or menstruation. Killing oneself is not easy; success requires careful planning. Women in the premenstrual phase show a marked tendency to be careless, thoughtless, unpunctual, forgetful and absent-minded. This inefficiency at a time when they are more likely to try to end their lives may result in a disproportionate failure."

Every suicidal gesture should be taken seriously, as a sufferer's mood may deteriorate so suddenly just before or during menstruation that an attempt may be made at a most unexpected moment. The attempt may end the life, even though it was only intended as a cry for help, or it may result in some permanent damage even harder to cope with than the premenstrual complaint. Drug overdoses may result in permanent liver or kidney damage, and when a woman throws herself under a train or from a high window, the scarred face and broken limbs are ever-present reminders of the condition which made life so intolerable. One patient produced her diaries with a record of 40 overdose attempts. Each one had needed hospital admission and had occurred during her premenstruum, those four fateful days before menstruation.

Edith, a 24-year-old personal assistant, wrote:

"On December 6th, realizing how dangerous the premenstrual effects were, I felt in great need of help. Unfortunately my group meeting was during this time and did not help me at all. After the meeting I rushed home, hid from my boyfriend whom I saw downtown, and intended again to overdose. Fortunately two friends arrived on the scene, and by the time they left it was all over and I had started to menstruate."

Depression can be an emotion, such as when we hear of the death of a near friend or other bad news, but it can also be an illness, when it affects all the bodily functions as well. The symptoms of a depressive illness are similar to premenstrual depression, but there are differences, one being in the timing. Whereas in a depressive illness the symptoms are present day after day throughout the entire month, and may last for weeks, months or years, in premenstrual depression the symptoms are measured in days and do not last longer than 14 days, for after menstruation the woman is her normal, happy, energetic self. Another important difference is the marked irritability which accompanies premenstrual depression. Premenstrual depression increases with age after 26 years and is common among single women.

Depression is best thought of as a disease of "loss," for there is a loss of happiness, interests and enthusiasm, loss of memory, energy, sleep and sexual arousal. One feels a loss of security and adequacy, and a loss of the powers of concentration, so that it becomes difficult to read a book or follow a television play. There is a loss of self-control, and an inability to make decisions or to control one's tears, behavior, and appetite. There is a loss of insight and an inability to realize, in the case of premenstrual depression, that very shortly the symptoms will pass and there will be a return to normality.

TIREDNESS

"What worries me most is that I get so slow and stupid before my periods." This comment by a journalist is echoed by many who find the lethargy, exhaustion, and prostration so difficult to cope with during the premenstruum. The "can't-be-bothered" attitude takes over and disrupts the program for the day, until in the end "everything goes."

Frances, a 32-year-old working mother, hated the tiredness most and wrote:

> "The worst and most worrying symptom is the feeling of apathy which descends on me; all physical and mental activity becomes a real effort and all I want to do is curl up in a corner away from everyone and all my responsibilities. I find it quite frightening that I cannot think clearly or quickly, and feel mentally dulled. These symptoms get increasingly worse and a couple of days before a period I feel quite ill. The first day of a period I feel a bit headachy and tired, but then it is like a weight being lifted off me and for two weeks or so I feel really fine."

Again, the tiredness may vary in severity from the typist who fills her wastebasket with her typing errors to the executive who feels unable to compose letters and stares all day at a blank sheet of paper. A mother of two boys, aged one and three, wrote:

> "When I am bad I stay in bed all day. One day last holiday I felt so bad I could not bear to lift my sons or get them dressed, so the poor children had to stay in bed the whole day. I just cried and told them how sorry I was

that I could not help them at all. I fear the little ones who have known me like this may grow up into disturbed children, but I promise you I'm quite normal at other times in my cycle."

One woman, as yet unknown to me, asked for an appointment, and when describing her tiredness added:

"I seem to be in a daze on those days, can't do anything right — more than once I've crossed the road to go to the restroom and found myself in the Men's room."

Another housewife confessed that:

"Just before a period, for about ten days, a sleepiness takes me over and all I want to do is sit down and sleep, so therefore no housework or proper cooking gets done."

It is the premenstrual tiredness which is responsible for the drop in mental ability before menstruation. At one boarding school it was possible to study 1,561 weekly grades of schoolchildren and compare them with the previous week's grades. Each grade covered the total scores of some seven to 12 different subjects. During the premenstrual week there was an average drop of 10% compared with a compensatory rise of 20% during the week immediately following menstruation, as shown in Figure 9. This effect is also evident in high school and college level examination results.

IRRITABILITY

It is those who are nearest to a sufferer of premenstrual irritability that suffer most, and this is usually not only the nearest but also the dearest, which means the husband, children, or parents. As one wife said:

"Pity those around me when the least things upset me. I hate everyone, shouting and picking quarrels, and the whole world gets on my nerves and I can only look at it with a jaundiced eye."

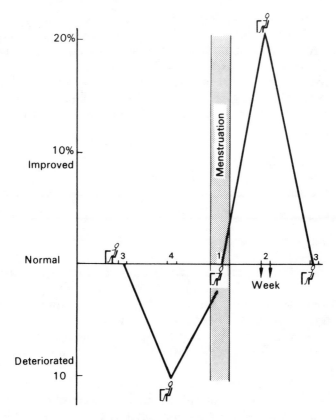

Figure 9 Variation in schoolgirls' weekly grades with menstruation

Premenstrual irritability is more common in the married woman, and the husband naturally has problems trying to calm a supersensitive, edgy, irrational, and agitated woman during these days of each cycle. Too many cases end up with visits to the marriage guidance counselor or in divorce.

The following three quotations taken from letters received suggest that the husband has obviously suffered as much as his wife:

"I have been suffering from premenstrual tension for some years now, and recently it came to its height. In July I was in my usual depressed state and, being angry, I didn't know what to do with myself; I just lost my temper and for the thousandth time I kicked the door and required forty stitches in my leg. My husband is at his wits' end, not knowing what to do with me, not knowing what I'm going to do next, and is ready to leave me after being married only eighteen months. I keep telling him that I'll be good the next time, but I never am and just can't control myself."

"Last Saturday I deliberately smashed all the dishes after clearing the table. I started menstruating in the evening. My general practitioner puts it down to my Irish temper. I get so depressed, hateful, horrid, tired, stay in bed, shout, and I could go on and on like this. It is my husband who asked me to write for help."

"At thirty-two, there is very little hope for me except the change; I have a history of suicide attempts, child and husband bashing, and many fights with a long-suffering doctor, who has been accused by me of many crimes, neglect and attempted manslaughter amongst them; at my worst I have taken many prescribed anti-depressants in massive overdoses."

If one sees a patient shortly after an aggressive outburst, like those described above, it is possible to get full details of the time at which food has been taken during the day. It is a common finding that the irritability is always worse when, in addition to the closeness of menstruation, there has been a long interval since the last meal, causing the blood sugar level to fall (see the discussion on blood sugar levels in Chapter 16). When patients are asked at what time of day their irritability rockets, it is usually in the late morning if breakfast has been missed, or when preparing the evening meal or waiting for the husband's return if he is later than usual. Often the wife has only had a sandwich, or possibly just cheese and an apple at midday, and is then at her wits' end, having eaten nothing else in anticipation of the evening meal. These sudden explosive outbursts of irritability or aggression can usually be helped by ensuring that regular small meals are taken at intervals of three hours. In two recent cases of murder and one of infanticide, it was found that no food had been taken for nine hours.

At the height of the tension there may be true confusion with memory loss, so that the woman is unaware of her actions or surroundings. Indeed she may bitterly refute any action, for she has no memory of it. The following notes made by a patient show how extreme the confusion may be, and how it may well approach temporary insanity.

"From the 4th onwards severe depression with secretive confusion. On the 7th I planned to kill my mother and myself. I wrote suicide notes to all concerned and took certain prescribed drugs that I thought would work. I do not know whether I would have done it as my friend, with whom I have a good relationship, discovered that they were missing and flushed them down the toilet. It took quite a few days before I realized how bizarre the whole episode was. The loss of appetite, need for alcohol, aggression, lack of interest and swollen glands continued until menstruation started on the 9th. These notes are written on the 18th, when my mind is clear."

It is not surprising that premenstrual tension, with its irritability and confusion, frequently leads to brushes with the law. There are those cases of assault where in a sudden fit of temper the woman throws a rolling-pin at her neighbor, or a typewriter at her boss, or tries to bite off a policeman's ear. There are the cases of baby-battering, husband-hitting, and homicide, as seen in the cases already quoted. Becoming drunk and disorderly when under the influence of alcohol or drugs may also lead to charges of assault. In France it is recognized that premenstrual tension may be so acute and so violent as to be classed as "temporary insanity" in courts of law.

My British survey, in 1961, of 156 newly committed women prisoners, revealed that half had committed their crime during the paramenstruum, and that the premenstrual syndrome was present in two-thirds of these women who committed their crime during the paramenstruum. Theft accounted for the highest proportion, with 56% of crimes being committed during the paramenstruum, while the alcoholics charged with being "drunk and disorderly" were a close second at 54%. In the same women's prison twenty years later two psychiatrists, Dr. D'Orban and Joy Dalton (no relation to the author), confirmed these findings in relation to crimes of violence, finding 44% had committed their offense during the paramenstruum and 34% suffered from premenstrual syndrome.

The Parisian police noticed early this century that 84% of crimes of violence by women had been committed during the premenstruum or menstruation. This was confirmed by a similar study in New York which showed that 62% of crimes of violence occurred during the premenstruum.

Dr. Morton and his colleagues working in Westfield State Prison, Bedford Hills, New York, showed that it was worthwhile treating the inmates of prisons and reformatories if they suffered from the premenstrual syndrome. He found that treatment resulted in an increased work output, less punishment for disobeying rules, and an increase in general morale.

The question may well be asked here: What benefit will a woman gain from a prison sentence or fine if she is unable to control her premenstrual irritability or confusion? Unfortunately, these premenstrual syndrome prisoners, if untreated, usually serve their full sentences without remission for good conduct, because their symptoms get the better of them each premenstruum and cause further problems.

5

Waterlogged

For some women, the days from ovulation to menstruation are characterized by a gain in weight, with a feeling of bloatedness and heaviness. This is due to an accumulation of water in the tissues and cells of the body, because only part of all the water that is taken in during those two weeks is passed out, while some remains and gradually accumulates. Not only is water retained but so is sodium, while potassium is lost. It should be stressed that water-retention is only one of the many symptoms of premenstrual syndrome, and many women never experience it at all even though they may suffer from severe premenstrual tension or other symptoms.

The commonest sign of water being retained in the body is an increase of weight, which may average 4 to 7 lbs. above the normal weight, (Figure 10) but can be even more, as much as 10 to 12 lbs. The normal weight is that which is taken during the postmenstruum, and gains and losses of up to 3 lbs. are usually considered within normal limits for women. Dr. William Thomas of Chicago has documented a case of one woman who gained between 12 and 14 lbs. each premenstruum, and then lost it altogether with an excessive output of 9 pints of urine on the first day of menstruation, the excessive urine output continuing for the next few days. Those who regularly gain and lose very large amounts of water periodically are sometimes diagnosed as suffering from "cyclical idiopathic edema."

Early workers on the premenstrual syndrome believed that the amount of premenstrual weight gain was an index of the severity of premenstrual symptoms, but this is definitely not the case. Dr. Bruce and Professor Russell of Maudsley Hospital, London, examined 34 women who complained of pre-

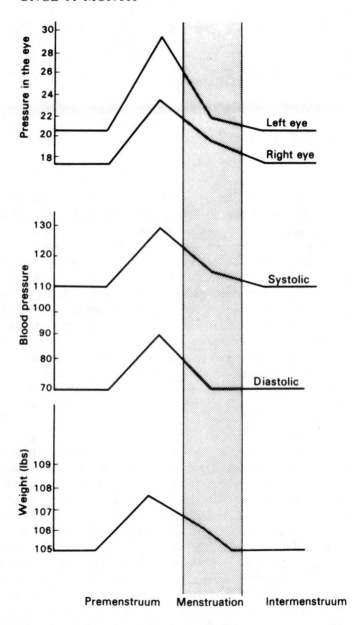

Figure 10   Fluctuations during the menstrual cycle in weight, blood pressure and pressure in the eye of a sufferer of premenstrual syndrome

menstrual symptoms, carefully measuring their weights and the amount of fluids they took in and the amount they passed out, and found no relationship. In fact, they wrongly concluded that the premenstrual syndrome was a purely psychological condition.

Apart from the gain in weight, water retention shows itself in the different tissues, with varying effects, as experienced by *Gladys* who wrote:

"The pattern of 5 lbs. weight rise at period times makes me so bloated that it turns me out of my favorite slacks and makes me feel ready to burst. My breasts become enlarged and sore, needing a larger size bra, my eyes sink back, and I get dark rings under the eyes. There is extreme fatigue, both physical, so that I can hardly put one foot before the other, and mental, so that I feel incapable of dealing with the children I teach. I am subject to quite black depressions caused by trivial things going wrong. I get throbbing and severe headaches in the week preceding the period, and always during the first three days of bleeding. I do a full-time job, look after the home and three children, go to evening classes, I also paint and do flower arranging, so you see I do try to fight it."

BREAST SORENESS

Complaints of breast soreness with enlargement and tender nipples are common, and all too frequently this leads to fears that this may be a sign of cancer of the breast. It is definitely not related to cancer in any way. It is more that the breast tissue is getting ready in the hope that following ovulation a pregnancy will occur, and the breasts will be needed for breast feeding, rather than as mere sex symbols. It must be emphasized that not all cases of breast tenderness are because of premenstrual syndrome, only those cases where cyclical soreness is present in the premenstruum with complete absence of pain after menstruation. Breast engorgement that is present throughout the month but more marked in the paramenstruum may be caused by an increased output from the pituitary gland of the hormone prolactin. It is possible to measure the blood prolactin level, and, if this is raised, treatment with bromocriptine may be beneficial.

FLUID RETENTION

The extra water in the tissues can cause ankles and fingers to swell, so that shoes have to be discarded and the wedding-ring removed. There may be swelling of the gums, so that dentures no longer fit. The skin coarsens and becomes blotchy, contact lenses won't fit, and the hair becomes lank. One model, who refused to accept work during the premenstruum, said:

> "I look my very worst, my skin won't take make-up, my face goes stiff, and I can't move gracefully with those extra pounds of weight!"

The exact place where the water accumulates varies in different women, and at different times in their life. The most severe symptoms result from water accumulating in a small unstretchable area, such as the labyrinth of the inner ear, which causes dizziness; when it enters the eyeball, causing raised pressure inside the eye and severe pain; and when it occurs inside the unyielding, bony skull, causing headaches. The sinuses are air spaces within the bones of the face where air enters through a small entrance which is lined with cells of the mucus membrane; when these are engorged and swollen, the entrance to the sinus is blocked, causing stale air to accumulate in the sinus and resulting in sinus headaches or "vacuum headaches." Water can also accumulate in the discs between the vertebrae of the spine, causing backache.

Sometimes there is a widespread distribution of the extra water, which produces vague symptoms in the muscles, joints and soft tissues, causing generalized rheumatic pains, abdominal bloating and heaviness. The water is always in the cells or in the fluid between the cells; it is never free, although one patient imagined she could hear the water "splashing within her abdomen." When the extra water accumulates in the fat and subcutaneous tissues there can be an appreciable gain in weight, without any other complaints. This is most likely to happen in obese women.

LOCATING THE WATER

The actual site where the cells become swollen may vary from time to time depending on such factors as (1) anatomical abnormality, (2) heredity, (3) injury, and (4) infection. Thus, a premenstrual sinus headache is more likely to occur in a woman whose cartilage in her nose is bent. Water is readily attracted to cells which have recently been injured or infected, so that after a fracture of the leg or arm it is usual to notice premenstrual swelling there for some months. If water retention occurs during the premenstruum in someone who has recently had pneumonia, it may cause a return of the cough or breathlessness.

This water retention is often blamed for the depression and other symptoms which accompany it. *Helen*, a 27-year-old unmarried accountant, wrote:

> "I start to get tender, swollen breasts, usually 14 days (ovulation?) before the beginning of menstruation, and I gain several pounds in weight. This makes me depressed and bad-tempered, and when you feel like that you can't help getting annoyed with everyone around you."

Many of the symptoms of water retention are characteristically worse in the early morning, often waking the patient from her sleep. This is especially so with migraine and with the acute pain in the eyeball that mimics glaucoma; and asthma, when there is swelling of the lining cells of the small tubes of the lung. Some people are awakened by a feeling of pins and needles, and perhaps numbness of their fingers. This is because the nerve passes from the arm through a narrow bony tunnel at the wrist, and when the surrounding cells are swollen and waterlogged this nerve becomes constricted. It is this which causes the odd sensations in the fingers, and it may be called "carpal tunnel syndrome."

Nowadays, many drugs are available which help to increase

the amount of urine passed, and these would seem to be a simple answer to the problem of water retention. Unfortunately, the problem is not quite so simple. Although these drugs or diuretics can get rid of water, extra water forms again quickly; it is rather like baling water from a boat with a hole in it. It is better to bung up the hole and prevent further water entering, than merely to keep baling. Just as the balers get tired, so do the water tablets. The temptation then is to use stronger and even stronger drugs to get rid of more and more water. But, as mentioned at the beginning of the chapter, the problem is not only that water accumulates but also that potassium is lost. Diuretics cause water and more potassium to pass in the urine, so unless sufficient potassium is added there may be a marked lowering of the blood potassium level, resulting in increased tiredness and possibly also weakness of the legs. Doctors can estimate the blood potassium level to know how much potassium is circulating in the blood at a given moment, but this does not indicate how much potassium is actually present in the cells, or in the fluid between the cells, which is what really matters.

Another problem is that water retention does not cause premenstrual tension, depression, tiredness or irritability, so none of these symptoms will be relieved by diuretics. Actually, diuretics are useful only in the short term until progesterone treatment can be given, or in mild cases where it can be used sparingly with the addition of extra potassium if blood tests show this is needed.

Several patients who have received diuretics continuously for many years may have become dehydrated. If the diuretics are stopped suddenly, these patients complain bitterly, within a day or two, of feeling bloated. They need to be persuaded to gradually tail off their diuretics by using them every other day, starting immediately after menstruation. After a month or two it may be possible to decrease the dose to every third or fourth day, until it is only used when the weight gain is really marked.

When a woman starts to gain weight there is the very natural temptation to start dieting. If her weight is above the ideal weight for her age and height this can be beneficial, but she needs to be careful which diet she chooses. Not for her a diet of fruit juice and liquids only, as this will merely increase the water retention. If she tries to solve the problem by missing meals she risks the possibility of her blood sugar level dropping abnormally low, thus increasing the depression and irritability. Dr. Jerome W. Conn of Michigan was the first to describe, in 1955, a condition of primary aldosteronism, known as Conn's syndrome. He probably knows more than anyone about water, salt and potassium balance, and he has suggested that the body's reaction to a low blood sugar level is related to the amount of potassium in the cells. He has shown that the blood sugar level can be improved by correcting the potassium deficiency which may be present.

On the other hand, if a woman is already below or at the average weight for her height and age, it is important for her to appreciate that the weight gain is due to excess water, and she should try to limit her fluid intake to four cups daily and restrict salt, rather than try to count calories and restrict her food.

6

Monthly Headaches

Many women like to jump on the bandwagon, and claim that their particular variety of headache only comes at period time. Undoubtedly, menstruation is the most frequent time for migraine attacks in women, as shown in Figure 11, in which the times of 935 migraine attacks are shown in relation to the days of the menstrual cycle. On the other hand, those who can produce a three-month record showing a regular and definite relationship of the headache to menstruation have a much better chance of obtaining relief from progesterone treatment. In Figure 12 it will be seen that Isobel's headaches last between 7 and 10 days before each period, and are preceded by symptoms of tension which ease off during menstruation. Joan presents a different picture: her headaches only last one or two days, and there is no premenstrual tension, but the headaches all tend to come around the time of menstruation. Kathleen seems to have headaches every 10 or 12 days; occasionally they coincide with menstruation, but often they just come at any time. It is unlikely that Kathleen will benefit from hormonal treatment.

Characteristically, monthly headaches which are likely to benefit from treatment with specific hormones, such as progesterone, are those which show a definite relationship to menstruation in a three-month record, and those headaches which started either at puberty, after a pregnancy, or while on the pill. These women are likely to be free from headaches after the fourth month of pregnancy, and may well look back to the later months of pregnancy as the only time in their life when they knew what that freedom was like. But alas, these same women are also likely to say that, immediately after the pregnancy, the headaches returned worse than ever.

Women who find their headaches becoming worse while they are on the pill, or who have a tendency to headaches on the first or second day after stopping the course of pills, are likely to be responsive to treatment. The majority of these women are also likely to find that after the menopause most of their problems come to an end.

The three common types of headaches related to menstruation are (1) sinus or vacuum headaches, (2) tension headaches, and (3) migraine.

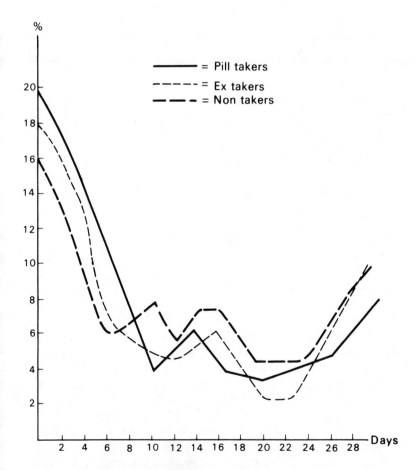

Figure 11 935 migraine attacks in relation to the menstrual chart

Isobel

	Jan.	Feb.	Mar.	Apr.
1	hT	hT	M	
2	hT	HT	M	
3	hT	HT	M	
4	nT	HM		
5	HT	M		
6	HT	M		
7	HT	M		T
8	HM	M		T
9	hM			T
10	hM			T
11	M		T	Th
12	M		T	Th
13	M		T	Th
14			Th	Th
15			Th	Th
16			Th	TH
17			Th	TH
18		T	Th	M
19		T	TH	M
20		T	TH	M
21		Th	H	M
22	T	Th	HM	
23	T	Th	HM	
24	T	HT	M	
25	nT	HM	M	
26	nT	hM	M	
27	hT	M		
28	hT	M		
29	hT			
30	hT			
31	nT			
Total				

Joan

	May.	Jun.	Jul.	Aug.
6				H
7				M
8				M
9			H	M
10	H			M
11	H	H	M	M
12	M	Mh	M	
13	M	M	M	
14	M	M	M	
15	M	M	M	
16	M	M		
17	M			

Kathleen

	Sep.	Oct.	Nov.	Dec.
1				M
2	H			
3			M	
4			M	
6			M	H
7		H		
11		M	H	
12			M	
13			M	
14	M			
15	M			
16	M			
22	H	H		
24				M
25				M
26				M
29			M	
30	H		M	

h = Mild headache   M = Menstruation

H = Severe headache   T = Tension

Figure 12　Headaches in relation to menstruation

VACUUM HEADACHES

It is better to speak of "vacuum headaches" rather than "sinus headaches," as the latter are likely to be confused with the headache resulting from true sinusitis, which is caused by infected material getting lodged in the sinuses. On the other hand, vacuum headaches are caused by the swelling of the cells at the entrance to the sinus, which block the entry so that stale air accumulates inside. These women generally know that a headache is on the way when their nasal passages become blocked and it is difficult to breathe through one nostril. There is tenderness or pressure over the sinuses, which are situated in the cheek bone and over the eyes. (Figure 13) The pain that results is made worse by bending

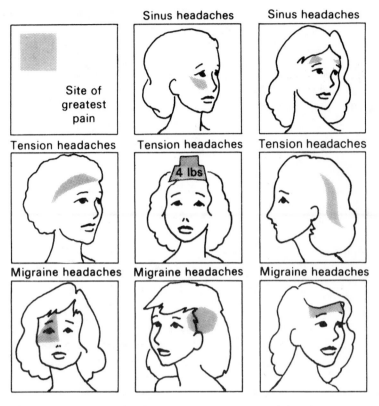

Figure 13 Sites of greatest pain in menstrual headaches

over, and may last from one to seven days. In addition, there may be other signs of waterlogging, such as a gain in weight, bloated abdomen, shortness of breath, or swollen ankles or fingers. These women would be wise to restrict their fluid intake to four cups of liquid daily, and may benefit from nasal decongestants.

TENSION HEADACHES

Tension headaches usually have a slow onset, so that a woman who is trying to chart her symptoms may be uncertain whether the pain in her head is bad enough to call a headache. A tension headache usually starts after symptoms of premenstrual tension — irritability, tiredness, or depression — and eases off gradually during the course of menstruation. The pain from tension headaches has been described as "like a steel band enclosing my head," or "like a heavy weight on top of my head." (Figure 13) These women will find that the usual analgesics such as aspirin or paracetamol will only give relief for about four hours, then the headache returns again and the analgesic must be repeated. Treatment with progesterone (see Chapter 19) is most valuable for this type of headache, and it also relieves the other symptoms of premenstrual syndrome.

MIGRAINE

Doctors like to divide migraines into two varieties: the classical, and the common type. In the classical variety the patient has a warning or "aura," which lasts for about 20 minutes before the onset of a severe headache. This aura may be sudden flashes of lights, brightly colored stars and stripes, or a patch of blindness; or there may be a sensation of pins and needles in the tongue, the side of the face or the hands and legs. Many people suffer both classical and common migraine at different times over the years. Common migraine has no aura, and begins gradually, increasing in severity. Both migraines may be accompanied by nausea or vomiting and extreme prostration, and usually last between 24 and 48 hours, although some unlucky women find they last even longer.

Most migraine sufferers have a family history, with a parent, brothers, sisters, uncles or aunts also suffering, so they start life with a predisposition to migraine. Nevertheless, there are those among them whose attacks are related to menstruation and can benefit from simple advice and possibly also from progesterone treatment.

In order to help women who have frequent or severe migraine attacks, it is helpful to have full details of all they have been doing, and of the times at which any foods have been consumed. In practice an attack form, like that shown in Figure 14, proves valuable, and helps to isolate an individual trigger factor. The trigger factor is the last straw, which decides exactly when a migraine is going to occur in a susceptible woman. It is often the result of either going too long without food, so that there is a drop in the blood sugar level, or eating foods to which the sufferer is sensitive.

Name............................   Date...............................
                                          Day of week.......................
                                          Time of onset ....
                                          Duration ....
Day of cycle.......................   Days before next menstruation......

During the 24 hours *before* an attack:—

(1) Did you have any special worry, overwork or shock?
(2) What had you done during the day?
      Normal work?
      Unusual activity?
      Extra tired?
(3) What food had you eaten and when?
      Breakfast......................   Time..............................
      ....
      Mid-morning...................   Time..............................
      ....
      Lunch ....   Time..............................
      ....
      Mid-afternoon.................   Time..............................
      ....
      Supper ....   Time..............................
      ....
      Evening ....   Time..............................
      ....
      Bedtime ....   Time..............................
      ....

Figure 14   An attack form useful for isolating trigger
                factors in migraine

TOO LONG WITHOUT FOOD

When women are asked what sort of things start a migraine attack they often mention travel, theater-going, or the day after a special event for which they worked hard and prepared for several days: a garage sale, a wedding, or a special party. If the attack forms have been carefully filled in it is usually easy to spot if the migraine has been caused by too long an interval without food. Generally speaking, five hours between meals is long enough for most women leading a normal energetic life, but women with premenstrual syndrome will find that over three hours without food can be too long an interval. An overnight interval of 13 hours is usually considered the limit. After this length of time susceptible women, probably those already born with the tendency to migraine, will find they develop a headache. This explains why travel often causes a headache: with frequent interruptions and long distances traveled, meals are often delayed longer than usual. Similarly, if one is busy with preparations for special events, the food may all too easily be forgotten. And if you are giving the party, how easy it is to ensure that your guests have plenty to eat while you forget to take any food yourself.

Furthermore, one must consider not only the interval between meals, but the amount of energy expended during the interval. The more energy is exerted, the quicker the blood sugar level falls. Overnight fasting is often the cause of a migraine attack on waking, and there are those migraine sufferers who say they cannot sleep late on holidays or at the weekend because they wake up with a headache. Migraine is also likely to occur when the evening meal is followed by some energetic sport or a brisk walk, and no further food is taken before retiring to bed.

> An example of this was noted in a receptionist, who was also a keen skater, and normally had her evening meal at 6:30 P.M. On Thursdays she would be off to the rink for three hours of energetic enjoyment before retiring, but had no food after the evening meal. Every four to five weeks, she would wake with a migraine on Friday mornings. The attacks occurred during the paramenstruum, but were triggered off by the long interval without food and the energetic skating.

Full information about the effect of a drop in blood sugar level is given on pages 135–138. If the attack forms suggest that the woman has had too long an interval without food, or has been too energetic for the amount of food she has had, it would suggest that a sudden drop in blood sugar may have triggered the attack. The treatment then becomes obvious: avoid fasting, and remember to have an extra cookie with the morning and afternoon coffee or tea. Remember, too, that proteins such as meat, fish and eggs, will keep the blood sugar up longer, while glucose sweets only cause a short, sharp rise in blood sugar level followed by a quick drop, and thus provide only a temporary benefit.

FOODS CAUSING MIGRAINE

Other women whose migraine attacks are not caused by fasting may find that they are sensitive to certain foods, the commonest of which are cheese, chocolate, alcohol, and citrus fruits. A few are sensitive to ripe bananas, pork, onions, fish and gluten. In these cases the migraine attacks do not occur immediately after the specific food has been eaten, but some 12 to 36 hours later. This is because the attack occurs, not when the food is digested in the stomach, but rather when it is later broken down in the liver by the action of special chemicals known as "enzymes." It would seem that if one particular enzyme is not present, a wrong chemical action occurs, releasing substances capable of opening wide the blood vessels of the brain. These substances are known as "vaso-dilating amines," and two common ones are tyramine, which is present in cheese, and phenylethylamine, which is present in alcohol and chocolate; but there are many other vaso-dilating amines which can be formed by the wrong breakdown of everyday foods.

It seems that some women's sensitivity to vaso-dilating amines may be increased during the paramenstruum, so that although they are able to take small amounts of, say, cheese, after menstruation, as menstruation approaches or during menstruation even a minute amount is sufficient to provoke an attack.

Women who fall into this category would be wise to try and avoid the foods to which they are sensitive, remembering always that it is an individual problem. Foods which cause attacks in one individual will not necessarily cause attacks in another migraine sufferer. However, as mentioned earlier, there are often other members of the family who also suffer from migraine, so it may be worthwhile having a "gathering of the clan" at which all blood relations who suffer from migraine can exchange ideas about which foods they feel are detrimental to them. Often, a common food can be discovered to which all family members are sensitive.

Those who are sensitive to cheese will be happy to learn that tyramine is not present in cream or cottage cheese, but only develops on maturing, so among the particular cheeses to be avoided are Stilton, Cheddar, Parmesan and processed cheeses. However, they should be aware that mature cheese is often hidden in quiches, Mornay sauce and Italian dishes.

Red wine, sherry, port and champagne are probably the worst alcohols for causing migraine, but it is often possible to take a single glass of white wine with food without any after-effects. It is also worth considering the difference between grape and grain alcohols, for more people are sensitive to grape alcohols than to the grain alcohols like beer and whiskey.

Chocolate is often added to rich fruit cakes or finger cakes to give a good color, and to coffee dishes to increase the flavor, so those who are sensitive to chocolate should be on their guard. Plain dark chocolate is more likely to provoke an attack than milk chocolate. And how easy it is for those sensitive to citrus fruits to forget that this also includes mandarins and tangerines.

7

Recurrent Problems

My interest in the premenstrual syndrome was first aroused within a few days of qualifying as a doctor, and whilst working as a fill-in for a general practitioner. In the early hours of the morning a call was received from a 34-year-old mother of three children, who had an acute attack of asthma. The husband, who opened the door, was most apologetic for calling the doctor out at such an hour, but added, "Unfortunately it happens every month except when she's pregnant." The woman certainly had a severe asthmatic attack, and was quickly given an injection to ease her breathing. As I was driving home, the husband's words recalled my own migraine, which also occurred once a month, just before menstruation, and reminded me that the only times of freedom had been during my pregnancies. A visit to the patient later that day revealed that her first attack of asthma had occurred at the age of 17 years, coinciding with her first period, and she had had an attack of asthma with each menstruation thereafter. The medical textbooks did not mention this possibility, but Dr. Raymond Greene, who had helped me with my migraine, suggested that this patient should also be treated with progesterone.

In the early years it was essentially the bodily ailments which were noticed, with less appreciation of the tension and other psychological symptoms. A survey in 1982 of 1,095 women being treated with progesterone for premenstrual syndrome, when compared with the symptoms reported in the first article in the British Medical Journal in 1953 of women being similarly treated, emphasizes the differences:

	1953	1982
Headache	69%	33%
Depression	6%	35%
Vertigo	13%	3%
Skin lesions	13%	3%
Bloatedness	6%	31%
Asthma	5%	1%
Epilepsy	5%	1%
Breast tenderness	2%	21%

The only way to identify a chronic recurring symptom as being part of the premenstrual syndrome is to chart it carefully, together with the dates of menstruation, for at least three months. If this was done more frequently there would be many more women whose asthma, epilepsy, migraine, and a host of other complaints would be identified as menstrually related, and they would then be eligible for relief by progesterone therapy. At present the list of symptoms which can be related to premenstrual syndrome is almost endless, and certainly covers all the systems of the body. This means that almost all specialists, no matter what their discipline, are likely to come across its effects. In fact many of these symptoms are among the commonest that the specialist is called upon to treat. For instance, the neurologist sees most patients with headaches and epilepsy, the dermatologist sees many patients with acne and boils, the urologist sees patients with cystitis and urethritis, and so on.

Women with bodily, or somatic, symptoms related to menstruation will have the usual characteristics of the premenstrual syndrome, and they will have the onset at puberty, after pregnancy or use of the pill, or when menstruation resumes after a few months absence. They will be free from symptoms in later pregnancy, and symptoms will be eased after the menopause. There will be a high number whose symptoms start after a pregnancy complicated by pre-eclamptic toxemia, postnatal depression, or sterilization.

While it will never be possible to give a list of all the possible symptoms which may occur in premenstrual syndrome, the common ones can be discussed. (Figure 15)

Premenstrual ASTHMA appears to be caused by water retention in the cells lining the smaller tubes of the lung, which become swollen and prevent the free entry of air into the minute air sacs. Thus the cause is not necessarily allergic, in fact these patients may not respond to sodium cromoglycate (Intal) inhalers, as do those whose asthma has a definite allergic basis. Premenstrual asthma is particularly common in women in their thirties and forties. Usually, the women will volunteer that their attacks are brought on by stress and tension, but that may be because they have not yet related it to premenstrual tension. In the special asthma clinics in hospitals it is usual to find that about one-third of all women of childbearing age have menstrually related asthma. Two women, aged 18 and 42, who have been treated at the Premenstrual Syndrome Clinic, University College Hospital, London, had a record of over 20 admissions to intensive care units for acute asthma, until an alert ward sister noticed that the attacks always occurred premenstrually. Both have since become free from asthma after receiving progesterone treatment.

One of the most satisfying experiences is to be able to diagnose and treat a woman with premenstrual EPILEPSY. can be treated with progesterone and freed from all anticonvulsant tablets, with their many and unpleasant side effects. Furthermore, in Britain, if they are not taking anticonvulsant drugs and have been three years without an epileptic fit, they have the joy of having their driving licenses returned to them. It seems that premenstrual epilepsy is often a culminating symptom which follows gradually increasing tension and headache, so these patients do have a warning that an attack is imminent. There may also be marked weight gain, but this is not always the case. Often the final trigger factor that precipitates the attack is a long interval without food.

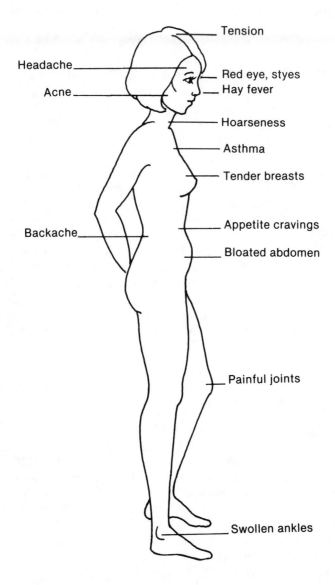

Figure 15   Common symptoms of premenstrual syndrome

Name __MARGARET__

	Jan.	Feb.	Mar.	Apr.	May	Jun.
1		M				
2						
3	X					
4						
5	M					M
6	M					M
7	M				M	M
8	M				M	M
9	M				M	M
10					M	
11					M	
12					M	
13						
14						
15				M		
16				M		
17				M		
18				MX		
19			M	M		
20			M	M		
21		X	M	M		
22			M			
23		M	M			
24		M	M			
25		M				
26		M				
27		M				
28	M			*		
29	M					
30	MX					
31	M					
Total						

Margaret is 27 yrs old with 2 children, onset after 1st pregnancy

Name __NANCY__

	Jan.	Feb.	Mar.	Apr.	May	Jun.	Jul.
1							
2							
3			X				
4				X			
5				M			
6			MX	M			
7			M	MX			
8			M	M			
9		X	MX	M			
10							
11		X					
12			M				
13	M	MX					
14	M	M					M
15	M	M					M
16	M	M				M	M
17	M	M				M	M
18	M	MX				M	
19	M	M				M	
20	M					M	
21						M	
22							
23							
24							
25							
26							
27							
28							
29					*		
30							
31							
Total							

Nancy is 28 yrs old, onset at puberty

M = menstruation
X = epileptic attack
* = progesterone treatment started

Figure 16 Charts of two patients with premenstrual epilepsy

Laura, 28 years, with one child, set off on holiday having had only a light breakfast at 8 A.M. Her husband drove some 300 miles, stopping only to ask the way. When she arrived at her hotel she had a nasty headache, and while she was unpacking, at about 5 P.M, she had an epileptic fit. She started menstruating the next day. She later agreed that there had been mounting tension during the previous week, which she had attributed to trying to finish all the necessary jobs in time for her holiday.

The charts of two epileptic patients, Margaret and Nancy, are shown in Figure 16; both responded completely to progesterone treatment and both had their driving licenses restored.

RHINITIS or *HAYFEVER* is often mistaken for the COM-MON COLD. It is usual to hear women in April saying, "Do you know, this is the fourth cold I've had since Christmas," when in fact it is a premenstrual rhinitis occurring with the fourth menstruation since Christmas. Once it is recognized as a premenstrual symptom then the demand for antibiotics disappears. The rhinitis is due to extra water causing swelling of the cells of the nasal passages. If the swelling of the cells occurs a little lower down in the larynx it can cause *hoarseness*, which is a special nuisance to opera singers. One opera singer carefully arranged her singing engagements so that they avoided her premenstruum. Another remarked that during the premenstruum the quality of her voice changed, and she was unable to reach the high notes. This was corrected by progesterone therapy.

The *LOSS OF A SENSE OF SMELL* is probably more common than generally appreciated, and is presumably due to extra water accumulating in the cells that are responsible for the sense of smell. The manufacturer of a special brand of anti-perspirant/deodorant noticed that women tended to change their brand after three or four weeks use, complaining that it had ceased to function effectively. Market research showed that the dissatisfaction of the women was due to a premenstrual increase in perspiration and vaginal discharge, and a diminishing perception of the reassuring perfume of the anti-perspirant/deodorant product. This had led women falsely to believe that the product had lost its efficiency.

DIZZINESS or *VERTIGO* is a common complaint. In some surveys it occurred in a third of all sufferers of pre-menstrual syndrome. It is most frequent among those who have had children and are approaching the menopause. The dizziness gets worse if the woman bends over, and it may accompany a headache. The probable cause is excess fluid in the labyrinth of the ear, which is responsible for balance.

Similarly, *FAINTING* is common just before menstruation, and is most likely to occur when there has been a long interval without food, or prolonged standing. In England it is common among teenage schoolgirls who have missed their breakfast and have to stand for a long time at the early morning school assembly.

CYSTITIS and URETHRITIS are common symptoms during the premenstruum, and may be caused by the increase in vaginal discharge and generalized pelvic congestion.

JOINT and MUSCLE PAINS may come back each month just before menstruation, last only a few days, and then disappear without treatment. There may also be stiffness on waking in the morning, although this disappears within the hour. The pain is probably caused by localized swelling of the cells, or failure of muscle relaxation during the time of premenstrual tension. The water retention that accompanies many of these symptoms led to the mistaken theory that premenstrual syndrome was due to water retention, and could therefore by corrected by diurectics. The effect of such treatment has already been discussed.

There are many factors responsible for the formation of VARICOSE VEINS, including a tendency within the family. However, when they first begin to appear they may only be visible in the premenstruum, and later they may be painful only at this time of the cycle.

BOILS, STYES and ACNE are all common skin lesions, which frequently recur each cycle just before menstruation. Acne is perhaps a special case. It is caused by the grease (or sebum) being too thick and too plentiful. This grease is produced by sebaceous glands in the skin, and is excreted through the pores. If the grease is too thick it blocks the pores and causes acne. The skin only starts making grease, or sebum, at puberty, so in the first few years of its production there is often either too much, or it is too thick or too thin. Gradually, the body learns to make the right amount. Estrogen helps to slow down the production of grease, so acne often returns at the time of falling estrogen levels, such as at ovulation and before menstruation. This also explains why acne usually improves during pregnancy, when there is plenty of estrogen, and also in some women who are on the high dosage estrogen pill.

CONJUNCTIVITIS, or red eye, may return each month due to causes other than infection. It is interesting that the association of conjunctivitis and menstruation was known as long ago as the sixteenth century.

GLAUCOMA is caused by raised pressure within the eyeball. This may be due to a narrowing of the opening through which the circulating fluid in the eyeball drains away, so it is not surprising to find that when there is water retention during the premenstruum there may be an excess accumulation of fluid within the eye and also difficulty in draining it away. (Figure 10) When this happens the pressure within the eye is raised, which becomes very painful and, by pressure on the optic nerve, may interfere with the sight. A survey of patients of menstruating age with closed angle glaucoma (where the draining opening is blocked) at the Institute of Ophthalmology, London, revealed that 89% suffered from premenstrual syndrome. *Uveitis* and *Iritis* are two other troublesome eye conditions which tend to flare up premenstrually and which respond to progesterone treatment.

CAPRICIOUS APPETITE, FOOD CRAVINGS & BINGES occurring at the height of premenstrual tension and water retention are well recognized. However great the self-control may be during the rest of the month, there come those days when a woman is just "overtaken by a demon and eats enough for a week in just one meal."
Olive wrote:

"My life swings between cycles of feasting and fasting. Having lived on a careful diet of only 750 calories for two weeks and lost 4 lbs., I had an uncontrollable urge, which got me out of bed. I raided mother's pantry and ate two loaves of bread with peanut butter, a packet of ginger cookies, and an apple tart."

Doctors Smith and Sauder from McMaster University, Canada, studied 300 nurses and confirmed that the craving for food and sweets, and the desire to eat compulsively, occurred during the times of premenstrual depression.

The actual foods chosen when there is a compulsive eating session are invariably carbohydrates and sweets, suggesting that the body's natural defense is coming into action to prevent a too severe or prolonged drop in blood sugar level (see Chapter 16).

ALCOHOLIC BOUTS may be a feature of the paramenstruum. A survey of American female alcoholics revealed that 67% related their drinking to the menstrual cycle and were able to abstain at other times; they all felt that their drinking habits had either started or increased during the premenstruum. During the paramenstruum the process of breaking down the alcohol appears to be slowed, so that more accumulates in the bloodstream. Many women find they cannot hold their normal amount of alcohol at this time, which is unfortunate, as it implies that care is needed when using alcohol as a pick-me-up to relieve the depression and tension.

Dentists recognize that ULCERS IN THE MOUTH commonly recur during the premenstruum, and these are sometimes accompanied by ulcers in the vulva, vagina and anus. Most opticians have learned that when making appointments for fitting contact lenses they must consider the time of the client's cycle; fitting may prove troublesome during the premenstruum. Similarly, hairdressers know that if a perm hasn't taken, the chances are that it was done on the wrong day of the month.

DRUG REACTIONS are often reported during the premenstruum, and it always proves difficult to know exactly if they were caused by the drug or are a symptom of the premenstruum. This can also produce confusion when doctors are doing controlled tests of new drugs. Often one finds the dummy tablet is effective, whereas the real drug causes headaches, increased drowsiness, or nausea. But it may be because the dummy tablet is being taken during the postmenstrual week, when the woman is feeling well, and the real tablet during the premenstruum when she is just reporting her normal premenstrual symptoms.

Mention should also be made of pain known as MIT-TELSCHMERZ, or middle pain, which may occur at the time of ovulation. This is usually a mild, cramping pain in the lower abdomen, on one side or the other, usually alternating month by month. It accompanies the release of the egg cell from the ovary, and is possibly caused by the contractions of the tubes as the egg cell makes its way down to the womb. The pain only lasts a few hours, and may be accompanied by a vaginal discharge or even slight bleeding. Young girls are apt to mistake it for acute appendicitis, and more than one teenager has arrived at my office complete with a packed case so that she could be sent straight off to the hospital. In fact, there is no vomiting, no distention of the abdomen, and none of the usual signs of guarding and localization of pain which doctors normally look for when they examine an abdomen. It is important to get these girls to record the time of abdominal pain as well as the dates of menstruation, so that they themselves can appreciate the relationship. Although ovulation occurs alternately on the right and left side, it is not completely regular. For instance, it may be right, right, left, right, left, left ... so that at the end of the year it will probably have occurred an equal number of times on both sides. This pain, or sensation, should be regarded as Nature's signal that ovulation is occurring, indicating a favorable time for intercourse to those seeking to conceive, or a time for abstinence for those wishing to avoid a pregnancy.

8

Pain and Periods

A very welcome and much needed breeze of common sense has recently been wafted through the medical and gynecological fields by Drs. Jean and John Lennane, a husband and wife team who, in a well-reasoned paper on a group of disorders including period pain, point out that there is no justification for the old idea that "it is all in the mind." Indeed, all the scientific evidence that exists points toward a hormonal imbalance being the cause. They use a number of quotations from current medical textbooks which, they suggest, have led to an irrational and ineffective approach to the treatment of such disorders. These quotations included the following:

> "It is generally acknowledged that this condition is much more frequent in the 'highly-strung', nervous or neurotic female than in her more stable sister."

> "Faulty outlook ... leading to an exaggeration of minor discomfort ... may even be an excuse for not doing something that is disliked."

> "The pain is always secondary to an emotional problem."

> "Very little can be done for a patient who prefers to use menstrual symptoms as a monthly refuge from responsibility and effort."

The idea that period pains, or dysmenorrhea, are purely psychological was put forward because there were no abnormalities to be detected on full physical or gynecological examination, nor are there any suitable tests of hormone levels which can distinguish those who suffer once a month. However, gradually it is being realized that dysmenorrhea is due to an imbalance of hormones.

There are two quite different, and indeed opposite, types of dysmenorrhea, and as the treatment of the two types is different, it is essential to distinguish between them. There is *spasmodic dysmenorrhea*, which is characterized by spasms of abdominal pain, and *congestive dysmenorrhea*, in which there is congestion of water or rather water retention. This latter type has all the characteristics of the premenstrual syndrome, with the addition of period pains.

SPASMODIC DYSMENORRHEA

When menstruation first starts at puberty no ovulation occurs, nor is there any period pain; however, about two years later ovulation commences, and then spasmodic dysmenorrhea also begins. Often, at the beginning, ovulation does not occur every month but only on alternate months, so period pains only occur on alternate months. Spasmodic dysmenorrhea is most frequent between the ages of 15 and 25 years. It ends abruptly after a full term pregnancy, or it may gradually end with each period becoming less painful during the early twenties. The girl usually feels very well during the premenstruum, and then is suddenly doubled up with severe spasms of pain in the lower abdomen on the first day of menstruation. The pains are colicky in nature, coming about every 20 minutes and lasting about five minutes; in fact, they are similar to true labor pains. The girl obtains most relief by lying down curled up around a hot water bottle; aspirins may help take the edge off the pain, but gin is the old-fashioned remedy. The pain may be so severe that bed is the only refuge, and pain may continue throughout the night, preventing sleep. A monthly absence from work becomes the rule. The pain is easier on the second day and has passed by the third or fourth day. The distribution of pain is in the "bikini" area, as shown in Figure 17; in fact it covers the area served by the uterine and ovarian nerves. The severity of the pain continues relentlessly month by month and is not affected by stress. It may be helped, temporarily at least, by an operation popularly known as a "D&C," or a dilatation and curettage, used to stretch the opening of the womb. The girl is often immature, with sparse hair in her armpits and lower abdomen, small breasts with pink nipples, and acne.

It would seem that spasmodic dysmenorrhea is caused by there being insufficient estrogen for maturing and stretching the muscles of the womb. During pregnancy there is abundance of estrogen from the placenta for a full nine months; also, the muscle wall of the womb is stretched by the unborn babe. As a result, this type of period pain usually ends after pregnancy, and it is only on rare occasions that the woman subsequently suffers from premenstrual syndrome, so there are some compensations.

Sufferers of spasmodic dysmenorrhea are often advised to take more exercise or, alternatively, to relax more. While doing a survey for the British consumer magazine *"Which?"*

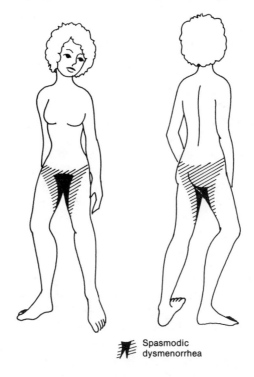

Spasmodic
dysmenorrhea

Figure 17 Site of pain in spasmodic dysmenorrhea

some years ago, over 200 women with spasmodic dysmenorrhea kept a careful record of the pain they suffered for
at least three cycles. It happened that the survey took place
in the summer, when many went on holiday. Some women
normally had active jobs, like waitresses or nurses, and they
tended to choose restful holidays lying in the sun. Others,
who had sedentary occupations, chose active holidays, cycling
500 miles, mountaineering and surfing. However, regardless
of their usual occupation or the amount of exercise they
took, the amount of pain experienced was unaffected by the
exercise or relaxation while on holiday.

A high level of another new hormone, called prostaglandin, has recently been found in sufferers from spasmodic dysmenorrhea; certain drugs known as prostaglandin inhibitors
are most effective in relieving this type of pain (see p. 173).

CONGESTIVE DYSMENORRHEA

Congestive dysmenorrhea is the presence of heavy, continuous lower abdominal pain during the last seven days of
the premenstruum, which increases in severity on the first
day of menstruation and then gradually ceases, together with
the end of the other premenstrual symptoms. The congestion
was thought to be due to water retention, but is now recognized as another presentation of the premenstrual syndrome.
In contrast to spasmodic dysmenorrhea, sufferers of the premenstrual syndrome may start with pain at their first menstruation and continue with it throughout their menstrual
life, and the symptoms are present whether ovulation occurs
or not. The pain is affected by stress, being worse when life
in general is in a turmoil and being eased by happy events. A
"D&C" brings no relief, nor does a pregnancy; in fact, premenstrual symptoms may become worse after each pregnancy.
Again, in contrast to spasmodic dysmenorrhea, the sufferers
of premenstrual syndrome are more mature and maternal,
with large breasts and brown nipples. An interesting fact is
that smoking tends to enhance the pain associated with premenstrual syndrome.

Estrogen administration increases the severity of the pre-menstrual syndrome, which responds positively to progesterone. Indeed, excess progesterone administered to girls who have not borne children can cause spasmodic dysmenorrhea. Thus, in theory, either type of dysmenorrhea can be produced at will by overdosing with the wrong hormone, estrogen or progesterone, which in itself proves that painful periods are not psychological but are caused by hormonal imbalance.

While stressing the benefit which can be obtained from appropriate treatment of painful periods, the very exceptional woman who does not ask for relief should not be forgotten. A 19-year-old filing clerk, living in a slum dwelling in a suburb in East London, was visited on one occasion for 'flu. In conversation her mother mentioned that she also suffered from severe period pains each month, and would be brought home from the West End in a taxi. My immediate response was that suffering of this caliber was no longer necessary today, whereupon the girl replied, "Oh don't! How else could I get a taxi ride once a month?"

MISPLACED CELLS

A rare cause of painful periods, which may come on with the first menstruation or after years of normal menstruation, and which affects only about one woman in 20 who has dysmenorrhea, is due to a condition know as *endometriosis*. Cells of the lining of the cavity of the womb, or endometrium, become displaced, and may be found either in the muscle wall or outer coat of the womb itself, or in the ligaments around the womb or ovary, or anywhere in the lower abdomen. (Figure 18 shows the relative position of the organs around the womb.) These cells lining the cavity of the womb have a unique ability to multiply, be shed, grow again, and multiply in an endless cycle under the influence of the menstrual hormones. Each time the lining cells are shed, they pass out from the opening of the womb into the vagina and out of the body as a menstrual flow. However, the misplaced cells are not able to pass out of the body, and instead tend to accumulate as tiny cysts, which later become covered with scar tissue. Each time thickening of the lining occurs during the premenstruum these cysts become larger, and as the cells are shed at menstruation more room has to be found within these cysts for the extra cells. So you can well imagine that after a time it becomes a very painful condition, with pain not limited only to the bikini area but spread all over the

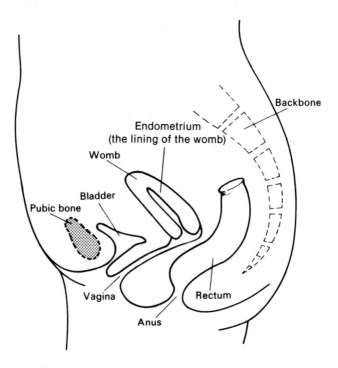

Figure 18   The position of organs around the womb

lower abdomen, possibly also affecting the bladder and rectum. In addition to painful periods, endometriosis is characterized by extreme pain during thrusting at intercourse, which may diminish and stop all sexual desire, and also by infertility due to scar tissue forming around the ovaries and tubes. Doctors can diagnose the condition by the story of painful periods, pain at intercourse, and infertility, and also by gynecological examination and if necessary by laparascopy, an operation in which a minute periscope is inserted through a small cut in the abdominal wall and the surgeon can then see for himself the tiny cysts and surrounding scar tissue.

Why the cells become displaced remains a mystery. It is possible that some were displaced during the developmental stage of the reproductive system in early fetal life, while it is also possible that some lining cells find their way through the fallopian tubes into the pelvis either at menstruation or labor. The pain is absent during pregnancy when there is no menstruation, although, as already mentioned, pregnancy does not often occur. The condition may be treated by stopping periods entirely for nine months or longer with hormone treatment. This not only stops menstruation, but also stops the cyclical changes in the normal and displaced endometrial cells. Alternatively, the abnormal tissue and cysts may be surgically removed or burned away by laser treatment.

9

Awkward Adolescent

The menarche, or first menstruation, is an important milestone in any girl's life, and demonstrates that she has an intact hormonal pathway from the hypothalamus and pituitary to the ovaries and womb. It is heralded over a period of some two years by the development of secondary sex characteristics, such as breast development, skin and circulatory changes, the growth of pubic and armpit hair, and changes of the body shape into the rounded female figure. (Figure 19) However, it is not the end of pubertal development, and only represents about the halfway stage.

The changes in the breast occur very slowly, from the first development of a small "bud" under the nipple the size of a grape, through the gradual increase in size to full development. Often one breast develops slightly before the other, but although this discrepancy often causes so much worry that immediate medical advice is sought, there is no cause for alarm. In due course both breasts will develop equally, for the growth stimulus comes from hormones in the bloodstream.

In India and Sri Lanka the first menstruation is a cause for celebration, as it represents the girl's attainment of physical maturity and the beginning of her sexual and reproductive life.The occasion is marked by a change from wearing short dresses to dressing in colorful and beautiful saris. There are reports that in Pakistan the girls in some households are deliberately fed on a low-protein diet in order to delay the menarche, thus postponing the cost of the marriage which is expected to occur immediately after the menarche has taken place.

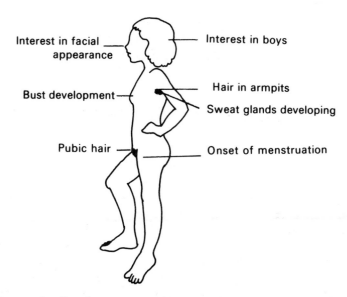

Interest in facial appearance

Interest in boys

Bust development

Hair in armpits

Sweat glands developing

Pubic hair

Onset of menstruation

Figure 19 Development at puberty

The attitude taken towards this pubertal development depends very much on the culture of the society to which a girl belongs. In some societies, such as Japan and Hong Kong, where the subject is still taboo, the girls obtain their information about their changes furtively, from the pages of the popular press. On the other hand, in America today sex education is discussed so freely at home, at school, and on the media, that when the menarche occurs it is almost a non-event. In any culture, however, the only girl in a male-dominated family may be especially fearful of the menarche because it emphasizes the many differences between herself and her brothers, and may increase the conflict over her developing femininity.

The age of the menarche is influenced by racial, genetic, dietetic, social, and economic factors. In Britain and the U.S. the average age of the menarche is 13.1 years, but it varies throughout the world, being highest in the Bundi tribe in New Guinea at 18.8 years and lowest in Cuba at 12.4 years. There is an early menarcheal age among British children attending special schools for the deaf and blind, where menarche occurs at the average age of 12.2 years, and an even earlier menarcheal age among those with congenital abnormalities that are known to start in early fetal life, like spina bifida and rubella. On the other hand, the mentally disabled and those with Down's syndrome tend to have a later menarche. The age range for normal children is from 10 to 16 years — in fact, only one girl in a hundred has not started menstruating by the age of 16. There has been a trend for the age of menarche to decrease since 1850, when it was 17.5 years, and this decrease is attributed to better nutrition. It is thought that the age of menarche has stabilized in the last 25 years.

The first menstruation usually lasts between three and eight days with an average of 5½ days, which is rather longer than most mothers expect it to be. Then there is usually an interval of two or three months before the next menstruation. Only about four menstruations occur during the first year after the menarche, with the cycle gradually becoming shorter.

Irregularity of periods is still quite frequent, and at the age of 16 years 20% of girls still have cycles which last longer than 40 days, and 33% have a prolonged bleeding lasting at least seven days. Irregularities of menstruation are quite common for teenagers and there are many quite normal reasons for this, but it can be very worrying for the girl herself. In these years she is not only adjusting to her developing feminine figure, she is also becoming more conscious of the opposite sex. As boyfriends come into the picture she becomes more interested in her own appearance and, all in all, these are often emotion-laden days.

In a single girl the cycle tends to be longer, perhaps 35 days, but as she begins to be stimulated by contact with boyfriends her cycle may shorten by a few days and approach the conventional norm, for the menstrual hormones are stimulated by male contact. However, if the male contact is broken, and she returns to female companionship, her cycle usually returns to its original pattern.

One 19-year-old inquired:

"My periods were always very irregular, with sometimes even eight weeks between them. When I first met John they became better, once as short as 28 days. Then we had an awful quarrel and I broke up with him. Since then, my cycles only seem to come when they want to, every five or six weeks. Does it matter?"

At 19 it does not matter, and probably even before she received a reply she would have found another boyfriend, and menstruation would have become more regular again.

About two years after the menarche ovulation occurs, not necessarily every month initially, but every two or three months, and gradually the cycles become more regular. It is with the onset of ovulation that spasmodic dysmenorrhea occurs. This usually comes as a surprise to both the girl and her mother, as previously menstruation had been so pain-free.

If spasmodic dysmenorrhea is bad enough to need regular medication to ease the pain, and especially if it causes the girl to take time off work or stay in bed, then medical help should be sought. It is interesting to listen to mothers explaining why they do not take their daughters to the doctor when they are suffering from spasmodic dysmenorrhea:

"I don't want to be considered fussy or neurotic."

"He will only tell her to get married and have children like I was told!"

"I would hate her to have an operation."

"He might put her on the pill; she's such a nice girl, besides she hasn't any boyfriends yet."

"Boys would take advantage of her if she were on the pill."

Such attitudes are a great shame, as there is so much that can be done for these girls. If the parents do not want their daughter to have the pill the doctor can always prescribe estrogen alone, which is not a contraceptive but will ease her monthly pains. Moreover, since the introduction of prostaglandin inhibitors, estrogen and the pill are no longer the only effective treatment.

Even before the onset of the first menstruation, cyclical mood swings may occur, and they continue even at times of missed menstruation. (Figure 6) These mood swings can transform a happy schoolgirl into a lazy, bad-tempered, selfish individual whose academic work and behavior deteriorate even before menstruation is established. As a pattern, it is very suggestive of the premenstrual syndrome, and events should be recorded so that help can be given to the girl before her work falls too far behind her schoolmates.

During these years, one may anticipate marked conflicts between the early maturers and those who mature more slowly. Firm friendships of several years standing may be broken as one develops and "fancies herself as a lady," and the other remains a mere schoolgirl. With maturation comes an interest in boys and an appreciation of feminine beauty, so that endless time is spent in caring for the face and body. At this time, grease starts developing in the skin and the sweat glands begin to operate, so that skin care and deodorants become necessary.

Many girls do not like the changes in body contour which Nature has decreed: they object to the rounded contours, and would prefer the broad shoulders and gawky limbs of boys. This stimulates the urge to diet, even in those who are not particularly overweight for their height and size. Excessive dieting during these developing years may halt menstruation and ovulation, and lead to *anorexia nervosa*. It is not unusual to find girls reducing their weight by strict dieting from 120 lbs. to 70 lbs. within a few months, and still complaining about their body and imagining that they are too fat. Unhappily, the road to recovery in such cases is slow and halting, and their future fertility is at stake; indeed, when menstruation does return, it is often accompanied by unpleasant premenstrual symptoms.

Unfortunately for most teenagers, this sexual development may be occurring at just the same time as their mothers are experiencing the difficult years of the menopause, and are also subject to mood swings and unpleasant symptoms. Nevertheless, it is important to help adolescents through this stage, however awkward, impossible and thoughtless they become. They should be given every opportunity to mix freely with both older girls and children, and with boys and men, to help them sort themselves out and appreciate the differences in individual men and women.

At puberty it is the premenstrual depression which is usually worse than the tiredness, and is likely to make a girl sullen, secretive, withdrawn, and anxious to be alone. Nevertheless, a careful watch should be kept on her behavior, as too often the mood swings occur suddenly, without warning or provocation, and she may make an unexpected suicide gesture.

Phyllis, 17 years old, had been at the top of her class at 12 years old, and her work was the envy of others. But she gradually went downhill in work and behavior. She became slovenly, rude, and bored with everything, gave up any attempt at graduating from high school, and left school at the first opportunity. She first worked in a hairdresser's shop, but her work was unsatisfactory and her time-keeping poor. Her next job was as a filing clerk, where her work was not appreciated. There would be days when she would come home, slip up to her bedroom and stay there for hours, allowing no one to enter and refusing food. One day her father found her apparently asleep in a corner, but the doctor diagnosed an overdose of hypnotics and arranged for her admission to the hospital for a stomach wash-out. This incident so shocked her mother that from then onward she kept a careful eye on her daughter. Soon the mother noted the correlation of awkwardness and menstruation, and asked for medical help. With treatment her daughter brightened up again, restarted her social life, which had been absent for five years, and later returned to evening classes, obtaining higher qualifications in shorthand and typing.

Girls with the premenstrual syndrome deserve treatment in their teens, and usually the need for progesterone is only temporary. Gradually, as they mature, the need for regular medication passes, although they may need it again in times of stress.

At one British boarding school, parents and visitors were invited to inspect the dormitories on the annual Open Day. On the mantel in each of the spotless dormitories was displayed a grade sheet, giving the grade each child had received for the tidiness of her bed and locker each morning. It was not difficult on inspecting these sheets to determine the menstrual patterns of the girls, for when they were exceptionally sleepy during the premenstruum they were more likely to receive a poor tidiness grade.

At another boarding school, punishment books were used to record the names of the girls, the date, and the reasons they were punished. These books were made available for analysis, together with the books the girls signed when they menstruated and needed sanitary protection. It was found that during menstruation the girls were twice as disobedient as would be expected. Many of the incidents during menstruation could be accounted for by tiredness, and included such offenses as forgetfulness and unpunctuality; others reflected the premenstrual irritability at having to conform to strict school discipline. In addition, a girl is more likely to be punished for an offense during menstruation because she may be too slow to avoid detection. If several children are all talking when the teacher enters the classroom, it will be those with a slow reaction time who will not stop talking quickly enough and will be caught.

This investigation also revealed two types of disobedience. When it had been completed the principal, an exceptional woman who knew and was concerned with each individual girl, was shown two lists of girls' names and asked to comment on them. Unknown to her, the lists contained the names of the girls who had received the most punishments during the term. One list contained the names of those whose punishments had all occurred during the premenstruum. "Just naughty girls from exuberance or laziness; I'll probably be choosing a future head girl from that list," she commented. But when shown the other list containing the names of girls whose punishments had occurred evenly throughout the menstrual cycle, she remarked, "They're the problem girls requiring careful handling and understanding," and she went on to describe how they had to cope with such difficulties as broken homes, foreign parents, or minor deformities.

In the study it was also noted that teachers' helpers, girls of 16–18, who were permitted to punish girls for misbehavior, gave significantly more punishments during their own menstruations, and then their standard gradually relaxed throughout the cycle. This naturally raises the question of the teachers, and indeed any women in charge, such as judges and supervisors: do they give more punishments during their own menstruation? Are they more strict then? Or, once they appreciate the effect of menstrual hormones on their behavior, do they bend over backward to try to avoid punishing too severely when they themselves are menstruating?

In this survey, it was also possible to analyze how many days passed before a girl who had been punished once was punished a second time, a statistical method known as "critical-event analysis." The results showed that most second punishments occurred within four days of the first offense, then fewer within five to eight days of the first offense, and then there was a gradual decrease in further punishments until 25–28 days after the first offense, when there was an unexpected rise not only in those girls who were already menstruating, but also in girls who had not yet started. This suggests that already these premenarche girls were experiencing mood swings, a fact that many observant mothers had noticed in their daughters. Incidentally, it was possible to do a similar analysis in respect of boys at a nearby boarding school, but they did not show any evidence of cyclical mood swings at all.

On one occasion my adolescent daughter burst into the house from school asking for a menstrual chart. When asked why, she replied that her teacher had lost her temper and thrown a piece of chalk at a girl, and the same thing had occurred on the Thursday before semester break, which was exactly four weeks earlier!

When my daughter left the twelfth grade she passed on to the next head girl of the school a list, compiled by the girls, of the probable dates of the teachers' menstruations, so that the girls would know when to hand in their essays to get good grades.

When, in later years, schoolgirls meet and exchange memories, it is the unfair incidents and unjustified punishments which are uppermost in their minds. One now wonders how often the blame could have been placed on it being the wrong day of the month for the teachers.

School principals have a dual responsibility: not only to cope with their own premenstrual mood swings, but also to recognize and deal with them in the girls for whose education they are responsible. They should be ready to step in with a kind word to girls who appear to have episodes of irritability or become depressed or disheartened, giving encouragement, particularly to prevent a girl from giving up a worthwhile career just because of some minor upsets or temporary difficulties.

As Figure 9 clearly showed, schoolgirls' work deteriorates during the premenstruum. A similar survey of women in the Armed Forces indicated lower intelligence scores in tests performed during the paramenstruum.

A study into the effect of menstruation on the results of high school and college level examinations showed that those girls taking examinations during the paramenstruum had fewer passes, less honors grades, and a lower average grade. The girls whose results were most affected during the paramenstruum were those with cycles exceeding 31 days, and those whose menstruation lasted for seven days or longer. In the high school examinations, some subjects were completed in one day, some had tests four days apart, and other subjects had tests at an interval of more than eight days. Consideration of the results in relation to the time intervals between exams on the same subject showed that girls were under greater handicap in those subjects where all tests were completed in one day, (when she could be in her paramenstruum) in comparison to subjects where exams were spaced more than eight days apart, in which case the girl could not have been entirely in her paramenstruum during both exams. It should not be difficult for examination boards and universities to arrange examination time-tables so that when two tests are necessary for a subject, they are eight or more days apart.

It might be mentioned that at public examinations in England, provision is usually made for proctors to make a note at the top of the examination paper of those candidates who are handicapped by the paramenstruum at the time of doing the exam. Of course, it is not known how much notice is taken of this fact by the examiners.

Another hazard is the increased sex desire which may occur premenstrually. This often takes over young adolescents, who are quite unprepared for this new sex urge and are unable to control their emotions. This nymphomanic urge may be responsible for young girls running away from home or custody, only to be found wandering in the park or following boys. These girls can be helped and their delinquent behavior abruptly ended with progesterone therapy.

10

Marriage

One wonders whether the cynic who wrote: "Marriages are made in heaven, but they end up in hell!" was married to a wife who had a severe case of premenstrual syndrome, or was just a keen observer of other people's marriages. Of course, not all marriages end up in hell, but for the young groom whose bride suffers from premenstrual syndrome or later develops it, the stakes run pretty high. Most men enter marriage sublimely ignorant of the problems women face each month; such knowledge as they have is probably confined to a vague awareness of "the curse" when she bleeds and is "on the rag." If their mothers or their sisters were sufferers, they might have learned how to cope with it, but the odds are that they are inclined to think that they were exceptional in their troubles, and they really know little about the cause.

While they were going out together before marriage, it may have been easy for the girl to hide her difficult days, and all too often it is not until they are living together that the truth begins to emerge. If she is a sufferer from spasmodic dysmenorrhea, he will be the first to see that she gets good and complete relief from her pains, for pain is something a man can understand. However, sudden mood changes, irrational behavior, and bursting into tears for no apparent reason may bewilder him, while sudden aggression and violence, when with little warning and no justification, his tender sweetheart unexpectedly becomes an angry, argumentative, shouting, abusive bitch, will shock and disturb him.

Fortunately, not all women suffer from premenstrual syndrome, nor do all premenstrual syndrome sufferers become hellcats. Even so, the husband-to-be should be made aware of the problem that can arise, how to recognize it when it first shows itself, and what treatment is available to provide complete relief. An article in the British magazine *Bride and Home* described what may lie ahead for the husband once the honeymoon is over:

> "Then quite suddenly you feel as if you can't cope anymore — everything seems too much trouble, the endless household chores, the everlasting planning of meals. For no apparent reason you rebel: 'Why should I do everything?' you ask yourself defiantly. 'I didn't have to do this before I was married. Why should I do it now?' Everything starts going wrong, and it gets worse instead of better.
>
> "As on other mornings, you get up and cook breakfast while your husband is in the bathroom. You climb wearily out of bed and trudge down the stairs, a vague feeling of resentment growing within you. The sound of cheerful whistling from upstairs only makes you feel a little more cross. Without any warning the toast starts to scorch, and the sausages, instead of happily sizzling in the pan, start spitting and spluttering furiously. Aghast, you rescue the toast, which by this time is beyond resurrection and fit only for the trash. The sausages are charred relics of their former selves and you throw those out too. Your unsuspecting husband opens the kitchen door expecting to find his breakfast ready and waiting, only to see a smoky atmosphere and a thoroughly overwrought wife. You are so dismayed at him finding you in such chaos that you just burst helplessly into tears."

What is the young husband going to make of such a situation? Much depends upon his family background. If he encountered similar situations at home before marriage, he will undoubtedly react as he did then, so that if he is used to making himself scarce and getting out of the house, he'll probably grab his bag and dash for the office, leaving her to sort out her troubles. If he was in the habit of helping to sort out the chaos, he'll probably sympathize with her, give her a kiss, make her a cup of coffee and breakfast, and insist on her going back to bed for the day. This latter is the wisest course of action.

But what if the young husband has never faced this sort of thing? How will he cope? Will he shrug it off, hoping that it is only a temporary lapse until, once a month, month after month it recurs? Or will he rage about breakfast being ruined and storm out of the house, to arrive at work hungry and unable to do his work properly, eventually returning home in a tired and frustrated state to an equally distraught wife? Not a happy augury for the future.

So far, in this chapter, we've been considering the state of the newlywed bride with premenstrual syndrome. There are those who don't start their symptoms until after a pregnancy. Just think of the situation. The couple have been enjoying an idyllic married life for a year or more, until the baby comes along, and now once a month there are the frustrations, mood swings, irritability, and apparent laziness — in addition to having to cope with the baby. From being the "blue-eyed boy," he now finds that he can do nothing right on those terrible days. If he has been an observant husband, and kept a diary of her menstrual dates, he will soon recognize the time relationship and, being sensible, will insist on her seeing a doctor and obtaining treatment for her premenstrual syndrome. On the other hand, if neither he nor she has any clear idea of her menstrual dates, they'll probably go on month after month until he can stand it no longer.

All this suffering is quite unnecessary, and a tragic destruction of family life. The answer lies in the true nature of marriage, which is that bride and groom, husband and wife, share equally in every aspect of their lives. If, when they are engaged, they both keep a chart of her menstruation and any symptoms that she may have, they will soon realize when things are going wrong; that is the time to seek medical advice and obtain treatment. If they keep the chart together, it will help them to understand each other better, and the fiancé, and later husband, will have a much greater understanding of what menstruation means to a woman. He will also find that he is the first to notice the warning signs of premenstrual syndrome, such as the slight irrationality of her conversation, or lack of conversation, the minor disagreements in which there is a certain rigidity in her views. More important still is the darkening of the skin around the eyes, one of the surest signs that she is about to enter her premenstruum. In some women the skin goes so dark as to appear almost black.

If at this time the fiancé or husband suggests that she should start her treatment, or go to the doctor, he will receive a flat denial that there is anything wrong. In fact she is quite unaware of the changes taking place, but this rigid refusal is another sure sign. If they have kept a chart together of her menstruation, this is the time to bring it out and check the cycle, when the time relationship should be confirmed. If she is already on progesterone therapy, the husband can then insist that she start using her progesterone suppositories or take some extra; if she is not undergoing treatment he should take her to the doctor together with the menstrual chart, or to a Premenstrual Syndrome Clinic if one is available. If treatment is not started at once, within 2–3 days she will be in the midst of her symptoms and it is then difficult to do much to help, for once the symptoms are manifesting, progesterone will not work. Progesterone must always be given *before* the symptoms start. All the husband can do in this case is to offer her sympathy, and assure her that he loves her — all of which will probably be rejected, but he must persist.

If there are children, he should remember that they are more likely to get out of hand with mother no longer able to care for and play with them. He must try to be a substitute mother as well as a father, and exercise his control over them. He should remember that there is housework to be done, and it is no use telling her to rest; he has to be practical. If the work has to be done and there is no one else to do it, she will not rest. A neighbor or a relative could be asked to help; it will probably only be for four or five days, unless the symptoms are very severe. Once menstruation has started, and while events are still fresh in their minds, he should impress upon her the need for medical help, and assure her that he will go with her. More husbands accompany their wives to the doctor or hospital when asking help for premenstrual syndrome than for any other gynecological condition, including infertility.

The following quotes from recent mail reveal how often the husband is involved with his wife's premenstrual syndrome:

"I am fortunate in having an extremely long-suffering husband who puts up with my tirades as best he knows how, but he says he doesn't know how to cope with me."

"My husband first noticed the connection with my menstrual cycle without mentioning it to me eighteen months ago, and backs me up completely in writing to you."

"The misery has gone on for years, misery and misery. Seventeen jobs in ten years. Now I clean offices, and for two weeks out of the month my husband gets up at 4 A.M. and does them for me."

Not uncommonly, the husbands have devised their own means of confirming the diagnosis beforehand; thus the computer manager came complete with a computer print-out to prove it, while a draftsman turned up with a beautifully drawn blueprint; others merely bring along the office diary or kitchen calendar.

But there are still too many husbands who have not made the diagnosis, or, more rarely, do not realize that help is available. They may know when they wake up that it's one of those days and, no matter what they do, they will not be able to satisfy their wife. If he returns home with some red roses she'll ask, "Why didn't you bring me my favorite chocolates?" but when he brings the correct brand of chocolates it'll be, "You know I'm dieting, how very cruel of you." He just can't win.

The monthly problems may interfere with his social life and his earning capacity. Some years ago a door-to-door salesman was sent by his employer for medical help. He worked on a commission basis, and while his average weekly commission was quite high, in one week in four his earnings fell drastically. Not only did he find it difficult to plan his spending, but his chances of promotion were being affected. The salesman explained that he became more depressed and seemed to start work later during the weeks his earnings were low and could not explain why. When asked about his wife's menstruation, however, the significance gradually dawned on him. A few days later he brought along his wife's menstrual record, which confirmed the diagnosis. Her irritability and tiredness were hindering her husband. She was delighted to be offered progesterone treatment, and responded well. Her husband was also delighted when he got a promotion.

Marital disharmony is a recurring theme among those seeking medical help:

"My marriage broke up seven years ago, and I feel this trouble was a big cause of the break-up. I have since turned down a chance to remarry, as I cannot face burdening someone with my continual monthly ailments."

"This premenstrual misery is a very real threat to the survival of our marriage."

"We have been married for eight years, during which time my premenstrual tension has been a constant problem. During the past three years this has become more acute and increasingly more severe, with a traumatic effect on our relationship and with that of our two boys of five and three years."

"My husband has urged me to write; our marriage is breaking up, my children are suffering, and after five years of my trouble my poor husband can take no more."

"My husband has already left me, and I have two children who I try hard not to lose my temper with at this time, but I feel sorry for them; it is really awful."

"I have come to dread my periods, and even my husband rushes to the calendar at an unexpected outburst on my part. I get violent with my husband."

Sometimes the marital disharmony manifests as just silence, on other occasions there are vicious verbal battles, and, at the extreme limit, there are the fights and batterings. How many wives batter their husbands during their paramenstruum is unknown, nor do we know how often the husband is provoked beyond endurance and batters her.

One mother wrote about her daughter, who was receiving treatment for premenstrual irritability and food cravings:

> "Some cakes and cookies disappeared on Sunday. It was all too much for me and I burst into tears. This in turn upset my husband, who went and found Mary in her bedroom and gave her a good thrashing. At midnight we discovered she was missing. She had spent the night with friends. Both Mary and I started menstruating that day."

Here is a case of menstrual synchrony, with mother's and daughter's menstruation occurring at the same time, and where the mother's tears caused the fraught husband to beat his daughter.

Two researchers in Washington, D.C., Roger Langley and Richard Levy, have estimated that there are 12 million battered husbands in the United States. They reckon it is the "most unreported crime," affecting 20% of husbands. Again, one is just left wondering about the effect of the paramenstruum, how often were the wives also victims of their own hormonal imbalance?

A couple of quotes to suggest that the premenstruum may frequently be the cause:

> "I attacked him with a carving knife on one occasion, and while building a stone wall I lifted huge stones and hurled them at him."

> "I have tried to knife my husband too many times to count...but for one fantastic week I feel on top of the world."

Most marriage-guidance counselors are well versed in the traumas which can be caused to the marital relationship by premenstrual syndrome, and try to draw the partner's attention to this. Often, when telephoned urgently for help because of a massive quarrel, a wise counselor will arrange a meeting seven days later, when the woman is more likely to be in her rational postmenstrual phase, having more insight and being more amenable to reason.

While the housewife may be content for most of the month to cope with the cooking, cleaning, shopping, mending, ironing, and perhaps even the gardening, there may come one of those days when it all gets on top of her, when she's too apathetic to cope with everyday chores, when she burns the cooking and leaves the house untidy. Alternatively, she may have a spurt of restless energy, obsessively polishing all and sundry until she wears herself out and then blames her premenstrual symptoms on the fact that she "overdid it." One difficulty facing the housewife at home all day is the temptation to miss meals, waiting to enjoy a meal with her husband at night. During the paramenstruum she will face the problems of low blood sugar levels.

The working wife faces different problems. In her effort to control herself in front of her fellow workers, and possibly also the public, she holds back her frustrations until she reaches home, and then lets go at her nearest and dearest. Again, she may well have missed her lunch and gone a long interval without food, not appreciating the problems this causes.

An important problem the couple must face is that of sexual harmony. Dr. Ruth D'arcy Hart, Medical Officer at the Fertility and Problems Clinic in London, found that among married women 60% noted their sex urge was greatest before menstruation. Unfortunately for those with premenstrual syndrome, this is also the time at which many of them are most unapproachable to their husbands. It is the time when it is so easy for her to claim she's too tired or, out of anger, to refuse his sexual overtures. Incidentally, one of the side effects of the pill, too rarely mentioned, is its ability to decrease the natural sex urge. Satisfactory sex between partners is the best cement for any marriage. There is so much that can be done these days if difficulties develop in this side of marriage that it is really worthwhile seeking help. One cause of a decrease in sexual satisfaction, which has only recently been recognized but is most responsive to treatment, is a loss of sex urge occurring after a pregnancy complicated by postnatal depression. A blood test may show the wife to have a raised prolactin level, in which case treatment with bromocriptine can be effective.

Men do not have cycles akin to women. On page 81 a

"critical event analysis" is described which detected cycles of disobedience in premenarcheal girls. Similar analyses have been done on surveys of disciplinary incidents among prisoners and schoolboys, and symptoms of glaucoma in men and women. The results were similar except that there appeared to be a return of the critical event after an interval of 25–28 days in women but not in men.

Margaret Henderson of Australia has shown that men have an ovulation temperature chart which is synchronous with the wife's chart. When the wife has a mid-cycle temperature drop followed by a rise at ovulation, which then continues at a higher level until menstruation, the husband also has the sudden drop in temperature followed by a rise, but the temperature does not then stay up continuously. However, if the wife has an an ovular cycle, with no drop and rise at ovulation, the husband's chart follows suit and he does not show an ovular rise. If the wife goes on the pill or becomes pregnant, and so stops ovulating, again the husband does not have the characteristic drop and rise. If the man moves out to live alone, or with another man, again the characteristic drop and rise will be lost. All of which suggest that when a couple are in harmony together their bodies' rhythms become synchronous, the man taking the lead from the woman's cycle.

As mentioned earlier, a good proportion of husbands accompany their wives to the doctor's office if she is suffering from premenstrual syndrome, and the remainder will usually agree to come to the next interview. This is a most valuable opportunity to learn more about the full extent of the wife's problems. At the same time, there is much useful information which can be given to the husband to help him cope better with the situation. First, he must understand what premenstrual syndrome is and why it occurs. Second, he should appreciate which of his wife's symptoms can be helped, and which are not premenstrual but occur throughout the month and are therefore not likely to benefit from progesterone treatment. He should be taught how to chart the symptoms, and may like to keep his own chart of events. Often the husband is the first to appreciate that his wife could benefit from some extra progesterone, and it may be possible to give the couple permission to raise the dose when they jointly feel the need is there. The husband should also appreciate the problems of low blood sugar levels; that his wife will be worse if deprived of sleep; and that at times of water retention her alcohol consumption should be reduced.

If the husband fully understands the situation, he will be able to make the necessary adjustments to their life. Thus one husband, realizing his wife's irritability in the premenstruum, asked their bank manager to send their joint balance sheets on specified days so that they could discuss their financial arrangements calmly in her postmenstruum. During the premenstruum, when the wife has little insight, many decisions about stressful things such as moving, holidays and schools must either be taken by the husband or postponed for a week or so. If help is needed in the home it may be better to arrange this for the one special week of the month rather than the usual one day per week.

How much responsibility should a husband have for his wife's premenstrual violence? In addition to ensuring that his wife receives treatment from her doctor, and making provision for the care of the children and the home when she is at her most vulnerable time, does he have a responsibility for the protection of the public? Should he report her violence to some appropriate authority? And indeed, which is the appropriate authority? What are his responsibilities if her violence brings her to court in conflict with criminal law? Too often such cases are reported too late, when the woman is already in jail accused of assault, infanticide, or murder, and the husband in her defense produces disturbing stories of her cyclical problems. All these questions need serious consideration, for at the present time there are no clear guidelines available to help the unfortunate family in such desperate circumstances.

11

Mother

The mother is the lynchpin of the family. When her life becomes a misery each month because of the effects of premenstrual syndrome, the consequences affect the whole family: husband, babies, schoolchildren, and teenagers. Children, even infants of only a few months, are sensitive to changes in their mother's temperament, and because they cannot understand the reason, they react to it in their own peculiar way.

When you ask adult sufferers of the premenstrual syndrome if their mother also suffered in the same way, you are likely to get many positive — and some rather interesting — replies, such as:

> "We used to say, 'The dragon's on the warpath,' and we all knew what it meant. But it only lasted a day or two."

> "I remember my brother putting up a red flag outside the front door to warn us to be careful in our approach to mother."

Health visitors and social workers soon recognize when one of the mothers in their care is in her premenstruum. The usually tidy house is slovenly and disorganized, the carpets are littered with old clothes, dirty dishes sit on the kitchen table, and there is probably a burnt cake by the sink. Maybe the children went off to school late, and in yesterday's clothes, and the chances are that the meals will not be ready on time.

Although premenstrual syndrome may start at puberty, it

usually gets worse — or it can begin — after the children are born, especially if there has been any depression after childbirth. This was a recurring theme in many letters:

"Since the birth of my last child two years ago (I have five children), I have changed from being a perfectly normal housewife and mother to an unpredictable, bad-tempered person. During my period, my moods make me feel positively ill, especially my head. If only I could grow a new one, I say to my husband."

"I have had intervals of depression since the birth of my first child, so that I have never regained confidence in myself since then."

"After baby's birth I changed, and now I get an incredible amount of head pressure for a few days prior to the bleeding. It feels as though the top of my head is about to blow off with pressure. I spoke to my doctor about the possibility of me starting an early menopause, but he only smiled and said it was more likely premenstrual tension."

"I have a twenty-two-month-old son, and I cannot remember feeling like this before he was born. I do love him very much, but the poor little soul does have a terrible time when I shout at him and make him sob his heart out. I seem unable to stop, although I feel terrible about what I'm doing. It is almost as though I must be getting some sort of pleasure from it, and I feel very, very upset and guilty afterwards."

Dr. Christine Cooper, a pediatrician, has stated that children can also be psychologically damaged for life by verbal violence.

The sudden onset of irritability after the birth of a child may surprise many mothers, who did not experience it before. They suddenly find themselves becoming quick-tempered, and making totally irrational decisions. They become impatient with the children, not waiting for them to learn to dress or eat for themselves. They won't accept that "kids will be kids," and shout at them when they are romping about harmlessly, and then complain that the children won't behave. They are like the school teacher's helpers who expected a higher standard of discipline when they themselves were menstruating.

When a mother's got so much to do it's easy enough to miss out on meals, which always has the additional benefit of slimming. Unfortunately, her irritable and aggressive outbursts are likely to occur when her blood sugar level is at its lowest, which makes matters even worse.

> *Rose*, an intelligent, unmarried 24-year-old mother, had contacted the National Society for the Prevention of Cruelty to Children herself, as she feared she might harm her six-year-old son during her premenstruum. It was obvious from her story that she had been very near to damaging him. She then described the usual timetable for the day: "Getting up at 8 A.M. and having a meal of toast and coffee together, and then walking half a mile to his school, doing the shopping on the way home, then housework until it was time to fetch him from school at 3:30 P.M." This was the worst time of the day, and just before her periods she would feel aggressive as she met him; suddenly a surge of hatred would well up and if he didn't behave, this is the time he would be smacked.

In fact, Rose was describing how she became irritable with her son 7½ hours after her last meal, having been energetic during the interval. Her menstrual chart confirmed that she only lost her temper during the premenstruum, and since she started receiving treatment with progesterone and eating a midday meal she has been happier and trouble-free. Incidentally, she would mark in advance on her menstrual chart the days on which she had to exert extra self-control as she was so anxious to do all that was best for her son.

Two remarks often heard after successful treatment of these patients are, "Even my children behave better," and, "They don't shout so much nowadays."

Contraception often proves a problem for these mothers. Those with premenstrual syndrome are liable to have side effects on the pill. Intrauterine devices (IUDs) can cause increased estrogen production, resulting in heavy menstruation becoming even heavier. Unfortunately, tubal ligation, previously thought to be a convenient permanent solution, has been shown to reduce the blood progesterone level. If they are receiving progesterone, this can be used contraceptively, as discussed on page 187.

CHILDREN CANNOT UNDERSTAND

Children, who cannot understand their mother's mood swings, may react with the development of psychosomatic or bodily symptoms, such as a cough, running nose, endless crying, temper tantrums, or vomiting. In my general practice, when children were brought in with such complaints, the mother would be given a chart on which to record the dates of the child's symptoms and another one on which to record the dates of her own menstruation. When the mother returned with the charts after an interval of two or three months, it was surprising how often it was clearly shown that the child was reacting, with various ailments, to the mother's mood swings. A survey of 100 mothers visiting the doctor because their child had a cough or cold showed that 54% of the mothers were in their paramenstruum. The children who were brought during the mother's paramenstruum had a tendency to be under two years, only children, those with symptoms of less than 24-hours' duration, and those whose mothers were under 30 years of age. One girl was only nine months, yet her mother brought a chart showing that for each time she had menstruated in the previous three months, the child had developed a cough and runny nose.

A six-month-old girl with herpes (or shingles) on her knee was brought to the office by her mother, who had recurrent premenstrual herpes on her upper lip of several years' duration.

A further survey was carried out among children who were admitted as emergencies to the North Middlesex Hospital in London. The mothers of 100 children were interviewed, and the result was very similar; in fact, 49% of the mothers were in their paramenstruum on the day the child was admitted. Some were admitted because of an illness such as asthma, abdominal pain, or a temperature of unknown cause, while others had been injured in an accident. If the mother is accident-prone during her paramenstruum, the child she is looking after is also accident-prone. If a mother is tired during the paramenstruum, she may not notice little Johnny running toward an oncoming car or climbing a dangerous tree, and so even he will be in greater danger then.

> One day, a telephone call informed me that an 18-month-old boy had had a high temperature and a convulsion. This was the third convulsion at intervals of three to four weeks. Enquiry revealed that it was not related to the mother's menstrual cycle, but to his Nanny who had total care of the boy while his mother worked full time. There had been some trouble with Nanny the day before, and she had just given notice. The two previous convulsions had occurred at the time of Nanny's paramenstruum.

SIBLING JEALOUSY

Sometimes jealousy of a brother or sister is incorrectly diagnosed, when the real diagnosis is premenstrual syndrome in the mother.

> *Susan*, aged 30 years, had been very well during her second pregnancy, with plenty of energy so that she would take three-year-old David out each afternoon to play on the swings or kick a football in the nearby recreation park. She had an easy delivery of a much-wanted daughter, but afterward became so depressed that she needed psychiatric treatment. David had been dry since the age of sixteen months, but after his sister's birth he gradually started to wet the bed again, not every night, but in batches every few weeks. It seemed all too easy to blame it on jealousy of the new baby, but when the mother kept a careful record it showed that David's bedwetting was occurring during her premenstruum. The mother then agreed she "hadn't been the same" since the baby's birth, and had been too tired and busy to take David out for his usual playtime in the park.

BATTERED CHILDREN

The most tragic presentation of the premenstrual syndrome is when it reaches such severity that the mother, in a state of confusion and rage, batters her much-loved child. These mothers, contrary to popular belief, are women who really love their child. They have strong maternal feelings, but in a sudden moment of premenstrual irritability their control is lost, and they injure their darling child.

A social worker's report on a 35-year-old mother of two children reads:

> "During the last premenstruum her youngest daughter, aged 18 months, was screaming and would not stop. Patient was very irritated by this and picked her up and squeezed her — this started a circle of louder screaming and harder squeezing until patient 'heard something crack.' She was immediately frightened and threw the child on the floor and sat crying on the chair. When more composed, she examined Joan and took her to the doctor."

This type of injury to a child is not uncommon. Judging from the letters and confidences of patients, it suggests that the cases of baby-battering that come to light are only the tip of the iceberg.

> "Because I lost my temper and hit my eldest child when he was four, just before a period, I nearly had a complete nervous breakdown. Even though I feel much better now, my premenstrual tension remains, and from day 18 of the cycle until day 4 of my period I suffer from depression, temper, forgetfulness and dizziness."

> "It has got to a stage now that every month something the children do triggers me off. It is as though there is somebody inside saying terrible things. I blame my son and tell him I hate him, and hit him. Sometimes he gets out of my way quickly."

If the situation deteriorates the children may be taken into care, but this is a drastic step. One is left wondering about the aftereffects on the many slightly-battered children, those who are not spotted by the social services and are not helped. Does the unsettled, temperamental background of such a childhood leave any scars such as shyness or lack of confidence?

A woman who had been treated with progesterone for 17 years was asked if she would like to take part in a television commentary dealing with the premenstrual syndrome. She went home and explained to her family that she couldn't recall those far-off days. "By Jove — Dad and I will never be able to forget your vicious temper," was the comment from her daughter, now in her twenties.

A 35-year-old teacher married to the principal of a school stated:

> "For seven days during the premenstruum I become tense, irritable, shouting, weepy and tired, bloated with swelling of my legs and ankles, and with headaches over my eyes. I have two children and at those times when I am in an uncontrollable temper, I have hit them really hard."

She was successfully treated with progesterone for 12 months and has been free from symptoms since. She later wrote:

> "It has been a valuable experience — I would never have believed that an intelligent woman like me, with high morals and good education, could ever lose control of herself to such an extent that she would batter her children, for I love my children dearly. How utterly illogical it is that I personally should cause them permanent harm."

When the child reaches school, the teacher may notice that absences seem to be occurring at regular intervals. One 10-year-old girl was referred for treatment by her teacher, who noticed absences for a few days at the beginning of each month. The teacher, in fact, wondered if it was because of the girl's menstruation, but it transpired that her mother had recurrent premenstrual asthma requiring rest in bed, and the daughter was kept at home to answer the door.

TEENAGERS' REACTIONS

Playing truant from school may also occur, as in the case of one mother who wrote:

> "For days before a period starts I hate everyone and make the family's life a misery. My thirteen-year-old daughter will not go to school when I'm like this. She is frightened of what I will do, and cries when I start drinking."

Teenagers, both boys and girls, are quick enough to spot the changes in their mother and notice when she's "in one of those moods," or as one boy said, "our whole life revolves around Mom's periods."

The mother's problem is not helped when the daughter starts to menstruate if both periods occur together in synchrony. Many mothers, recognizing the problem in themselves, seek help for their daughter's premenstrual syndrome. They may feel that they've weathered the storm so far, and it won't be long before the end, but they are not prepared to let their daughters suffer as they have done.

Finally, all mothers, and fathers too, have the responsibility of seeing that their children get good sex education, and especially know about those problems which come back once a month.

12

The Worlds Workers

The cost to industry because of menstrual problems is high, and it is measured in millions of pounds, liras, kroners and dollars, as well as in terms of human misery, unhappiness and pain. It has been estimated to cost British industry 3% of its total wage bill, which may be compared with 3% in Italy, 5% in Sweden and 8% in the United States. The load is not spread evenly, for the industries which suffer the most are those employing large numbers of women, especially the clothing industry, light-engineering, transistor and assembly factories, and laundries. Texas Intruments, which employs women for the assembly of electrical components, finds that the average worker's normal production rate of 100 components per hour drops during the paramenstruum to 75 per hour.

Research studies have shown that during the paramenstruum there is a deterioration of arm and hand steadiness, which is an adverse factor among those whose work demands manual dexterity. One podiatrist complained that during the paramenstruum her hands get stiff and she finds skilled movements difficult. "If ever I do cut a patient, you can be sure it will be during those premenstrual days," she says. One wonders if the same ever applies to surgeons.

Absenteeism directly related to menstrual problems is generally caused by spasmodic dysmenorrhea, premenstrual migraine, and asthma, for, as one library assistant remarked, "you don't stay away from work merely because of your bad temper; instead you soldier on and cause chaos by misfiling, and you get yourself a bad name." The influence of menstrual illness during working hours was demonstrated in a survey at a light-engineering factory employing 3,500 women, and also in the branches of a department store employing 10,000 women. It showed that 45% of the 269 women surveyed who reported sick were in their paramenstruum. Dr. William Bickers and Maribelle Woods from the Medical College of Virginia noted as long ago as 1951 that 36% of women in their premenstrual week requested sedation during working hours.

A survey in four London hospitals showed that half of all emergency admissions of women to hospitals occurred during the premenstruum. This figure was the same for medical emergencies (like coronaries and strokes), for surgical admissions (like colic and appendicitis), for infectious fevers, and for admissions to psychiatric wards. Admissions for depression and suicides have been shown the world over to be the highest during the paramenstruum.

Accidents at work are another problem to industry, both the minor cuts and bruises, which are a waste of working time and are treated at the first aid station, and the serious ones which require admission to the hospital. Research at the U.S. Center for Safety Education showed that the 48 hours before the onset of menstruation are the most dangerous ones, when most accidents at work occur. In Germany, it was noted that apprentice tightrope walkers had most accidents in the premenstruum. In restaurants, it is recognized that the premenstrual clumsiness of waitresses accounts for an undue number of breakages.

The lowering of mental ability during the paramenstruum accounts for unnecessary typing errors, and more than one secretary has been referred for treatment when her boss could no longer put up with those few days in each month when letters had to be returned for retyping. Journalists, artists, and authors find this a problem too, lacking inspiration and waiting hopefully for a brainwave, which is more likely to come during the postmenstruum. Errors in billing, accounting, stocktaking and filing take longer to correct than to make, and again the incidence of mistakes is highest during the paramenstruum. Premenstrual irritability may show itself in bad-tempered service by salespeople, receptionists and waitresses, who are all in the public view. The problems of lowered judgment during the premenstruum must be considered by teachers, judges and executives, who need to be on their guard against making hasty and wrong decisions. One teacher wrote with honesty, "Every month there are one or two days when I am simply not worth the salary my employers pay me."

There are some specialized occupations which have their own particular hazards on premenstrual days, such as the hoarseness which affects opera and other professional singers. One musical comedy star in the 1930s would, with devastating regularity, come into the theater once a month surrounded by a powerful aroma of garlic, which preceded her wherever she went. "You see," she would explain, "It's this sore throat again, and garlic is the only thing that saves my voice." Sure enough, four days later she would once again be in magnificent voice, but whether it was the garlic or her postmenstruum that was responsible is a matter of guesswork. For artists in the theater the premenstrual syndrome is a very real problem. One great impresario/producer would always attend rehearsal wearing a top hat and smoking a cigar. On one occasion his leading lady was making a fuss and obviously in her premenstruum. The great man stood up in the center of the auditorium, ground his cigar to dust under his feet, and hurling his hat on the floor stamped on it crying out, "Woman! I don't know why I employ you, you drive me to distraction!" There was a pause and in a changed voice he went on, "But when you are well — you're magnificent!"

One wonders how many so called "prima donnas," with their reputation for throwing tantrums, were really only reacting to their premenstrual syndrome? For the members of the chorus, the showgirls and ballet dancers, it is always a question of whether the stage manager has enough experience to realize their problem and help them over the difficult days. Their symptoms of bloatedness and puffy eyes and skin are shared by models and movie stars, who often have a clause in their contracts forbidding filming during the paramenstruum. The lowered sensitivity to taste is a handicap to cooks, who may over-flavor the sauces and other foods. Nor must we forget the woman astronaut, Russia's Valentina Tereshkova, who in 1973 had to be brought down after only three days in space when she began to menstruate heavily in the zero gravity.

In Argentina, women are allowed under the Constitution

to take the necessary days off for their menstrual miseries, and in India wives have long had the privilege of being excused from housework, as it is believed that any food they prepare may be spoilt.

The site of an individual's premenstrual symptoms may be determined by her work. An investigation into the incidence of premenstrual syndrome was carried out in a light-engineering factory. About 20 women were interviewed in batches each day. Some days it was noted that the predominant symptom was premenstrual backache, and on other days, complaints of headaches were the most common. Later, it became clear that all the women in any one batch came from the same department and were doing the same kind of work. Those who spent their working hours bending over a workbench were more likely to complain of backache, while those employed sitting at a bench assembling minute electrical parts, a task needing considerable mental concentration, complained mostly of premenstrual headaches.

Texas Instruments found that women had less menstrual absenteeism when they worked from 2 P.M. to 10 P.M., compared with the other shifts of 6 A.M. to 2 P.M. and 8:30 A.M. to 5:30 P.M. Maybe this was because the woman who woke up feeling ill had more time to dose herself and recover from her problems. It is certainly a point worth considering for those who are given an option to choose their own working hours. Sufferers from premenstrual syndrome usually cope especially badly with night-shift work, which seems to be because the "diurnal clock," which regulates the cycle of sleep and wakefulness, is situated in the hypothalamus and easily disturbs the menstrual clock. This has been found to be a problem with nurses, especially those in training whose regulations demand a specified period of night work. Night work too often leads to upsets of the menstrual pattern and to depressive illnesses in sufferers of premenstrual syndrome.

Premenstrual syndrome can affect the chances of getting employment, holding down the job, receiving promotion, and losing it unnecessarily. The problems of some sufferers are shown in the following excerpts from letters:

"I cannot plan to go anywhere during these depressing times and I live in constant fear of losing my job, as I have to take time off each month with a real sick head-ache. My chances of promotion have been ruined because of this."

"I have recently given up my job unnecessarily and realized that it is ridiculous to let this condition ruin my whole life. Although I know the cause of my depressive feelings, I seem to be unable to think logically, and though I know I shall be fine again in a week's time I seem to get quite illogical and irrational at the same time."

"I am thirty-three years of age and have suffered from the premenstrual syndrome for the best part of my adult life. The symptoms are horrible depression, muddle-headed-ness, and feeling dead from the neck up. I recently took the totally unnecessary and very impulsive step of resign-ing from my post as a teacher of English. Of course it was just before my period that I took this drastic step. I am well-qualified and have been doing this now for seven years. To all other people I appear cheerful, calm and efficient, especially when a period is not on its way."

A specialized problem arose in the Ortho Pharmaceuticals oral contraceptive plant in Puerto Rico, where breast enlarge-ment was found among the men and menstrual disorders among the women. This occurred despite the strict pre-cautions taken in making the synthetic estrogens. These included hermetically sealed machines, air conditioning, res-pirators, and special protective clothing (even down to the underwear). The long-term effects of occupational exposure to estrogens are practically unknown, and there are no safety standards in force anywhere.

How can industry best cope with the financial burden caused by menstrual problems? Fortunately, most employers are supplying convenient restrooms where a woman can relax for a few hours, take something to ease her sufferings, and return to continue work for the rest of the day. The avail-ability of flexitime, by which each worker clocks herself in and out of work at times that suit her best, is a blessing to many women. They can accumulate a few hours in reserve so that when they are at their lowest they need not go to work for that day.

Perhaps industry should tackle the situation more seriously by educating its staff, especially personnel managers and supervisors, to recognize and fully understand the problems so that they can better deal with them. For example, women can be assigned to less skilled jobs such as packing and stacking during their vulnerable days, rather than remaining on tasks which are more complex and harder to remedy later, such as soldering or assembly.

Finally, treatment centers should be available, as these problems are not insoluble and can be treated. Such centers should be available either in hospitals or at places of employment.

13

Lady's Leisure

Even when a woman is off duty, away from office and house-work and just relaxing, the black cloud of once a month may still be with her. Which woman looking forward to a week-end's pleasure either on a yacht or up in the mountains, on a bicycle or down in the caves, wants to be bothered with menstrual problems? Fortunately, there's an answer for those women who are on the pill. They can be asked when they start their initial course, "Which day of the week would it be most convenient for you to menstruate?" As menstruation can be expected to occur within two days of stopping the course, it is not a very difficult calculation to decide on which day to begin. Admittedly, there are some who would find it more convenient to menstruate at the weekends, when their husband can take over some domestic tasks and care for the children.

SPORTS

The strenuous physical training and weight regulation de-manded of top athletes, ballet dancers and gymnasts all too often leads to missed periods or a complete absence of men-struation. This condition, known as amenorrhea, may last many months or even years at a time. It is the runners, rather than the cyclists or swimmers, who are most affected by amenorrhea. Although superficially it may seem beneficial to be without the hazards of menstruation or fear of preg-nancy, it is now appreciated that the attendant lack of estrogen can result in brittle bones, as in postmenopausal women, so they become prone to stress fractures, especially the metatarsal bones of the feet.

What about the other sporting activities in which women indulge? Those who enjoy a game of club tennis, golf or racquetball may well find that their performance deteriorates during the paramenstruum, for it has been found that this is the time when arm and hand steadiness is impaired, sharpness of vision declines, and there may be a slowing of movement because of extra weight and water retention. The menstrual influence on many top sportswomen may be less obvious, because they are able to maintain a steady standard without fluctuations in performance. However, research by the British Women's Amateur Athletics Association confirmed that top athletes gave their best performance during their postmenstruum, and in preparing for the 1976 Olympics they arranged a little menstrual engineering (adjusting the time of menstruation) so that the British athletes at least did not have to rely on Nature's roulette.

Dr. Ken Dyer of Adelaide, Australia, has produced some interesting figures showing that over the past 20 years women's top athletic performances have improved more than men's. This suggests that within the next three or four decades women could be running and swimming as well as men, certainly in the longer distance races. Women have determination and aggression and are especially suited to prolonged exertion; they have the striking example of the Canadian, Cynthia Nicolas, who in the summer of 1977 set a new world record for crossing the English Channel twice in 19 hours, 55 minutes, compared with the previous male record of 30 hours.

HOBBIES

Women have so many hobbies that it is difficult to cover them all. There are those women who enjoy dressmaking, but will avoid cutting a dress out of expensive material on the wrong day of the month, for fear of spoiling it. Others will hesitate to spend money on flowers at that time, as they find they cannot arrange them to perfection. Artists may well have difficulties and feel their inspiration is lost, and have to wait until their postmenstrual peak to resume their creative activity.

Intellectual games may be affected once a month, as the partner at bridge may have discovered or the opponent at chess or scrabble may well appreciate.

DRIVING HAZARDS

Driving is a leisure-time activity for many women: for some it may mean an active participation in car rallies, while for most it is a social journey or outing. In either case, there will be a menstrual handicap. A survey at four hospitals showed that half of all accident admissions of women occurred during those vital paramenstrual days. Indeed, among those involved in an accident the menstrual influence was equally present among the passengers or passive participants, as among the drivers, who are the active participants. In those few seconds which elapse between the car climbing the curb and before it hits a brick wall, the alert passenger may brace herself up and cover her head for protection, while the passenger in her paramenstruum may be too slow to take even these elementary precautions.

Driving is a complicated task, requiring the coordination of many skills which are lowered during the paramenstruum. Complicated and rapidly changing road situations demand instant reaction and good judgment, and if this is lowered there may be an increase in the braking distance. Alertness of hearing is decreased, so that a driver may not hear a warning siren. Impaired sharpness of vision and a lowered ability to judge shapes and sizes means that a woman may lose her normal precision in parking and reversing the car. She may become impatient of the slow driver ahead, or of an elderly person crossing the road in front of her. She may overtake irrationally on a blind curve or drive aggressively around a dangerous corner. She may fail to notice changing weather conditions, poor light, or alterations on the road surfaces. She may forget to fasten her safety belt, or follow other driving laws. Even as a pedestrian she is still vulnerable in her paramenstruum, and may cross the road without the usual precautions, while as a mother she may not be alert enough to protect her child from dangers on the road. Having said all that, perhaps one should add that women are considered better risks than men by the insurance companies: women are at risk only during the paramenstruum, but are much safer during the postmenstrual peak.

SHOPPING

The joys of a shopping spree may be marred during the paramenstruum. A woman may become an indecisive, hesitant shopper who tries on all the shoes in the shop, finds they won't fit because of her swollen feet, and leaves the shop empty-handed. She may buy some totally unwanted dresses, which don't fit and are the wrong color, and which she'll never wear. It is possible that her color sense and appreciation of shape and size deteriorate during this phase of the cycle. A few women even buy unnecessary and expensive items, like furs and jewelry, merely to annoy their husband. One can't help feeling sorry for the man who wrote:

> "I know it's the wrong day for my wife if I come home and find the kitchen loaded with fruit, anything up to ten pounds of apples, bananas and oranges. I know she'll be in a foul temper and ask me to put the children to bed. But at other times she's the best wife in the world."

There is the problem of women shoplifters, who are caught during the paramenstruum. While it is possible that they really are in a totally confused state and are unaware of what they are doing, it is also possible that they are habitual shoplifters, who were caught at a time when they were not sufficiently alert and did not take their usual precautions.

ENTERTAINMENTS

Social entertainments may not be all that successful during the paramenstruum. Cocktail parties too often require prolonged standing, which isn't fun for those with water retention. As one woman put it:

"I can always recognize fellow sufferers, as they also edge their way towards the walls to rest their legs."

Other problems related to this time of the month are described:

"My problem is about ten days before a period comes. I get uncontrollable fits of depression, which makes me hit rock bottom. If I am with a crowd of friends, I feel like I'm going to suffocate; it's a feeling that comes over me and I want to run out, and I do run out."

"I often have to entertain for my husband. I am a good cook, even if I say it myself. An excellent meal is ready, but when the first guest arrives I just burst into tears. It ruins my whole evening. I've learnt to arrange my dates after my period, but then my period is bound to be late!"

Nor can the theater bring pleasure to everyone, as one sufferer from premenstrual depression recalled:

"I remember sitting in the theater with tears rolling down my cheeks — squeezing my hands and saying to myself, 'NO — I mustn't, this is a comedy — everyone else is laughing.'"

The problems of alcohol intoxication are increased during the paramenstruum, so that a woman can never really let herself go without ending up in trouble. Some women can never take cannabis without suffering its worst effects; others can take it at most times of the month and enjoy the experience, but if they take it during the paramenstruum they develop delusions or hallucinations.

Some women have an uncontrollable urge to gamble during the premenstruum, whether it is on horses, cards, or bingo. One of my patient's addictions is gambling on slot machines; on some days of the month she is just spellbound by them and cannot stop. Realizing the cause of her habit, she tries to go out without any money at those times to help remove the temptation.

14

Crime and Premenstrual Syndrome

It was a surprising coincidence that on consecutive days, two women in different English cities appeared in court charged with murder. Both women had their charges reduced to manslaughter on the grounds of diminished responsibility caused by premenstrual syndrome. Although the circumstances of their offenses differed, the evidence presented in each case led to the same conclusion: the defendant was suffering from a severe case of premenstrual syndrome. Both cases had been very carefully researched, and presented incontrovertible evidence of longstanding, bizarre, cyclical behavior occurring in the premenstruum with normality of behavior in the postmenstruum. The important point to appreciate is that these were two extreme and exceptional cases; it does not mean that all sufferers of premenstrual syndrome are potential murderers, nor does it mean that all female murderers suffer from premenstrual syndrome.

When a plea of premenstrual syndrome is made in the courts, it is even more necessary than usual to ensure that it adheres to the strict definition. Thus, there must be evidence of recurrent symptoms, or earlier episodes of a similar loss of control, confusion, amnesia or violence in previous cycles, or at monthly intervals.

Such evidence might be found in diaries, medical records, police files or prison documents, which often give the precise dates of marital quarrels, physical violence, previous suicide attempts or other serious incidents. Indeed, one woman accused of manslaughter had 30 previous convictions occurring at cycles of 29.04 ± 1.47 days, and the documents revealed that while in prison she had made attempts at drowning, strangling, escaping, slashing her wrists, smashing windows and setting fire to the bed in her cell. These episodes had been meticulously recorded by the prison officer on duty, and were found to have occurred at intervals of 29.55 ± 1.45 days. Thus, the diagnosis did not rely on the woman's memory. A study of the prison records also revealed that she had been described as "pleasant and cooperative, but at times she loses her senses and can be quite impulsive," which suggests that there was a complete absence of destructive symptoms after menstruation.

An 18-year-old ballet dancer who was accused of arson successfully pleaded premenstrual syndrome as a mitigating factor and was released on probation. She had an excellent school record and her behavior had always been exemplary, until she started menstruating. Thereafter she appeared to change in character, and had several episodes of unusual and unexplained behavior. One day, she suddenly went into her bedroom and shaved off her blonde hair and eyebrows; on another occasion, she ran away from home and was later returned by the police after being found drunk and disorderly; once she burnt the bedroom curtains; another time, she overdosed herself with pain relievers and alcohol and was admitted to the hospital overnight; finally, she set fire to her father's house and was admitted to prison. While in prison, she attempted to set fire to the bed in her cell, and on another occasion, she attempted to strangle herself by tying one end of a sheet around her neck and the other end to the top of the window. It was her father who noticed from his diaries that his daughter's problems occurred about once a month. He was advised to produce proof that would show the precise dates on which the many curious happenings occurred. He did this by searching through the doctor's and hospital's files, and by checking the dates of insurance claims for the burnt curtains, the date on the check on which he bought his daughter a new wig, and the precise dates on which she misbehaved while in prison. Again, the many occurrences were shown to be coming in regular monthly cycles. Ultimately, the girl received progesterone treatment and is now a successful executive.

A similar story can be told of an unemployed girl who harassed the police with unnecessary emergency phone calls, which disrupted normal police work. She had earlier been put in a reform school for making such calls, but after being released she persisted with the same offense and was imprisoned. Again, her father was the one who noticed that the problems arose each month, and drew the lawyer's attention to the coincidences. In her case, it represented a cry for help, akin to other women whose cry for attention might be a suicide attempt or self-mutilation. She, too, responded to progesterone, and was released on probation. However, after she left prison the progesterone was not restarted, and she again began making unnecessary police phone calls. This time no mercy was shown, and she served a two-year sentence. That was six years ago; today on progesterone treatment her life has changed, and she is now working with the disabled.

These represent genuine cases of criminal behavior, resulting from a hormonal disease which responds to treatment. These women should rightly be freed, for they cannot be held responsible for their sudden unexpected loss of control. However, the genuine cases are few and far between. A far bigger problem has now arisen, and it is our duty to ensure that premenstrual syndrome is not made a universal defense. Already, cases have occurred in Britain where this has been tried. A woman on her first charge of shoplifting cannot make a claim of premenstrual syndrome without evidence that this is a recurrent offense. The mere coincidence of two car crashes or two speeding offenses occurring in the premenstruum is insufficient evidence of premenstrual syndrome. The public has a right to be protected by the knowledge that the defendant is receiving progesterone treatment and is unlikely to be a further danger. At a recent appeals trial in Britain, premenstrual syndrome was rejected as a defense in a case of murder, although it still stands as a "factor causing diminished responsibility" in capital charges, and as "a mitigating factor" in lesser charges.

For the correct diagnosis of premenstrual syndrome, the precise dates of menstruation and of the alleged crime are a prerequisite. Yet a clerk in a travel agency, accused of stealing travelers' checks worth $1,000 from her employer at some unknown date between August 1980 and April 1981, pleaded premenstrual syndrome. Not surprisingly, the plea failed and a jail sentence was imposed.

Some women who suffer greatly from premenstrual syndrome are needlessly incarcerated. They are deserving of our sympathy, and justice will not be served until all true sufferers of premenstrual syndrome are properly diagnosed and treated. The road to rehabilitaton after a prison sentence is long and hard. The interests of all women will best be served by increasing our diagnostic capacity, enabling us to distinguish the genuine sufferers from the many malingerers who try to jump on the bandwagon, and whose claims of premenstrual syndrome can never be substantiated.

The interested reader will find further discussion of this subject in Appendix I: PMS — The Need for Legal Guidelines and Accurate Diagnosis (p. 205).

15

The Hormonal Control

Some scientists believe that the body is governed by bio-rhythms, which include a physical rhythm of 23 days, a sensitivity or emotional rhythm of 28 days, and an intellectual rhythm of 33 days. These body cycles are not affected by life's events and repeat themselves so unchangingly that they can be worked out for any individual by anyone who can count, or by computer, if the hour and date of birth is known. Under no circumstances should the menstrual cycle be associated with biorhythms, for it is completely different. No matter how precisely you can pinpoint your hour and date of birth, it will not enable you, or anyone else, to work out when your menstrual cycle will begin, what its length will be, or anything at all about its pattern of ovulation and menstruation.

The menstrual cycle does not begin at birth. It is interrupted by pregnancy and breastfeeding, and is altered by life events such as illnesses, examinations, bereavement, happy times, sad events, and changes in environment. Furthermore, menstrual patterns show endless variations in duration of flow and quantity of blood lost, as well as in the length of cycle.

When teaching about the menstrual cycle it is most convenient to consider a 28-day cycle. It makes for simplicity, and is easier when describing the various changes that occur, such as ovulation on the fourteenth day. But we must not lose sight of the fact that women are all individuals and do not fit naturally into neat pigeonholes. Sometimes one is asked, "What is the right length of the menstrual cycle?" One might as well ask, "What is the right height for a woman?" All individuals are different; one meets many healthy normal women who menstruate about every 21 days, as well as those at the other extreme who only menstruate on average every 36 days. Both are quite normal, with fully effective reproductive systems. The cycle of 28 days is only an average for all women all over the world. Chiazze and his colleagues found that only 62% of women aged 15–19 years had a menstrual cycle between 25 and 31 days, with the proportion gradually increasing with age, so that between 35 and 39 years there were 86% with an almost conventional cycle.

It is said that Dr. Pinkus, the father of the Pill, decided over a cup of tea with the British endocrinologist, Peter Bishop, that 28 days would be a convenient time interval to allow withdrawal bleeding to occur in women on the pill. So it is that today there are millions of women with man-made cycles of 28 days. But they could just as easily have decided on 24 days or 30 days.

When women are asked the length of their cycle the frequent reply is, "Oh, I'm always late," meaning it is more than 28 days, or, "I'm quite regular," meaning, "I never have to get worried because I'm never over 28 days." Incidentally, the days of a cycle should always be counted from the first day of menstruation until the first day of the next menstruation. Confusion sometimes occurs because women count from the end of one period until the beginning of the next; they count only the days they are not bleeding.

The duration of menstrual flow also varies from cycle to cycle and from individual to individual. It may be as short as two days or go on as long as eight days, and still doctors would consider it normal and know that these women would be able to have children if this was their desire. The quantity of the menstrual flow or blood loss is also variable, and as few people are likely to see another person's flow there is bound to be considerable exaggeration in both directions. Some women will even say, "I had a really good period," which could be interpreted as meaning the loss was bright red; many women object to the scanty dark red, brown or black loss which sometimes comes with the pill. It is helpful to realize that menstrual bleeding comes from the minute blood vessels on the lining of the womb and not from any big blood vessels, so that if bleeding continues for a very long time it might cause anemia, but one can never actually bleed to death as one could from a wound in a limb.

THE MENSTRUAL CONTROLLING CENTER

In the opening chapter, the menstrual cycle was broken down into seven four-day phases of hormone activity. Each hormone change is carefully monitored by the menstrual controlling center, often referred to as the "menstrual clock," which is not situated in the womb where the action takes place but at a distance from it, low in the brain, in a part known as the "hypothalamus." (Figure 20) The hypothalamus itself controls or orchestrates many other functions, among them being the centers for the control of water balance, appetite, weight, mood and the day/night rhythm, so that if any of these is upset it will tend to affect the others. The

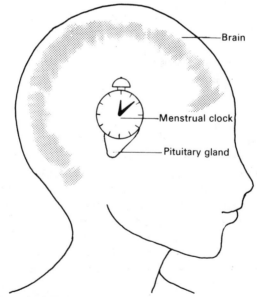

It is at the base of the brain in the Hypothalamus, above the Pituitary gland.

Figure 20   Position of the menstrual clock

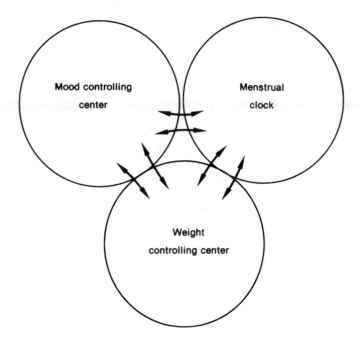

Figure 21   Diagram of controlling centers in the hypothalamus

diagram in Figure 21 shows the proximity of these centers,
which explains why, when the menstrual cycle is disturbed or
altered (such as by taking the pill), it can upset the weight,
the water balance and the mood centers, causing in turn a
gain in weight, water retention and depression. In a similar
way, if the appetite is drastically curtailed, as in anorexia nervosa, the menstrual cycle will stop and depression will develop. Again, depressive illnesses are likely to cause an
alteration in menstrual patterns, resulting either in excessive
bleeding, as in "weeping womb," or a break in menstruation.
It can also cause alterations in weight, either a gain or a
loss.

The diurnal controlling center, which is concerned with
sleep rhythms, is also situated in the hypothalamus, close to
the menstrual clock. Those with a sensitive menstrual clock
are likely to be easily upset by night shift work, and have
marked jet lag after long flights.

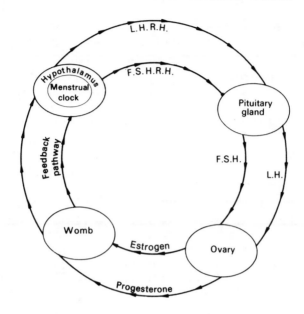

Figure 22 Menstrual hormonal pathways

MENSTRUAL CLOCK

The menstrual clock, being the control center of the menstrual cycle, is responsible for the smooth and effective operation of a woman's marvelous reproductive system. Situated in the hypothalamus, it has two hormones which it uses for this purpose. Hormones are chemical messengers with their own individual structure; they travel in the blood stream and are designed to act on a particular target organ. The two hormones that serve the menstrual clock have rather grand sounding names: Follicle Stimulating Hormone Releasing Hormone (FSHRH) and Luteinising Hormone Releasing Hormone (LHRH). Their target is the pituitary gland, which is situated next to the hypothalamus at the base of the brain. These two releasing hormones from the hypothalamus stimulate the pituitary gland to produce two other menstrual hormones, Follicle Stimulating Hormone (FSH) and Luteinising Hormone (LH), thus boosting the hormone output. (Figure 22)

The pituitary gland sends out a variety of different hormones which control, among other things, growth, pigmentation, lactation, thyroid functions, and adrenalin and insulin output. In short, it has a finger in every pie. But what concerns us now are the two pituitary hormones, follicle stimulating hormone and luteinising hormone, which act on the ovary. Follicle stimulating hormone acts on the ovaries to stimulate the formation of follicles, tiny microscopic rings of cells within which lies an immature ovum, or egg cell. As the follicles develop, specialized cells produce estrogen, yet another hormone, which is released into the blood stream. Estrogen builds up the lining of the womb, to replace the one which was shed at the last menstruation. But estrogen has another important function: before ovulation, it thins the cervical mucus, or natural vaginal discharge, to assist the sperms entering the womb in their search for the egg cell, which needs to be fertilized for pregnancy to occur. At puberty, estrogen is responsible for the development of the secondary sex characteristics, such as breast development, hair growth, and the rounded female contours.

At mid-cycle, it is the sudden surge of the other pituitary hormone, luteinising hormone, which causes the ripened follicle to burst and discharge its egg cell, a process known as "ovulation." Further stimulation by the luteinising hormone causes new cells to form at the site of the burst follicle, and these cells produce the other menstrual hormone, progesterone. Progesterone is secreted in spurts, and after ovulation it passes in the blood stream to its target organ, which is the womb. The levels of these hormones during a normal menstrual cycle were shown in Figure 1, Chapter 1.

After the lining of the womb has been rebuilt under the influence of estrogen, it is converted by progesterone into a soft, spongy tissue, hopefully ready for the embedding of a fertilized egg. Thus, progesterone is needed after ovulation, when the initial repair work on the lining of the womb has already taken place. Progesterone is also responsible for making the fallopian tubes contract more forcefully but less frequently, so that the egg cell may be swept along to the womb. Progesterone also changes the vaginal discharge from a thin watery fluid in which sperm could move freely into a thick sticky mucus, thus preventing further sperm from entering the womb. The presence of progesterone raises the body temperature again, in preparation for a possible pregnancy.

Nature has devised a magnificent machine in our reproductive system, complete with a highly efficient communication network between the hypothalamus, pituitary, ovary and womb, which is called the "feedback pathway." This ensures that the higher centers are kept fully informed of the progress down below (Figure 22) and can adjust the level of hormones according to the information received. For instance, should conception occur, the hormonal output is altered within hours. Another important control is prolactin, a hormone produced by the anterior pituitary gland which is involved in the progesterone feedback mechanism, so that if too much prolactin is produced the progesterone feedback pathway is interrupted.

OVULATION

Most women recognize when ovulation occurs, as there may be a slight sensation of discomfort for about an hour in one side of the lower abdomen. At the same time, they may notice that their normal vaginal discharge changes from a thin fluid to a thick, sticky mucus. Some women have a migraine at that time or a tendency to be irritable, while for the more unfortunate this may herald the onset of premenstrual syndrome. Sometimes, when the migraine or irritability at ovulation is severe, women have difficulty in becoming pregnant because they avoid having intercourse on the very days that they are most likely to conceive.

If a woman carefully records her temperature for two minutes every morning before getting out of bed it may be possible to decide whether or not she is ovulating, and also whether she has sufficient progesterone. In Figure 23 a few temperature charts are shown. *Teresa* is normal; ovulation occurred as shown by the sudden dip and subsequent rise in temperature until the start of menstruation. *Ursula's* chart is very steady and all on the same level, with no evidence of ovulation; it is known as an "anovular chart." *Victoria's* chart does show ovulation and a rise of temperature, but this rise is not maintained, suggesting that she has insufficient proges-

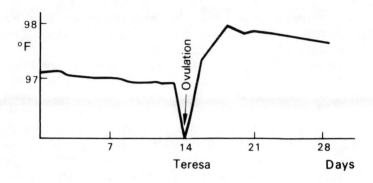

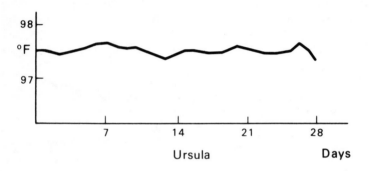

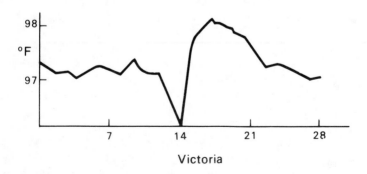

Figure 23   Temperature charts taken through the menstrual cycle

terone. It must be appreciated that temperature charts are not always reliable; ovulation can occur even with a chart like Ursula's.

The exact time of ovulation can be determined in several ways: by the change from a thin discharge to thick sticky mucus, from a daily temperature chart, using tests showing the time of the peak of luteinising hormone in the blood, and by direct inspection of the ovary either at the time of an abdominal operation or by laparascopy, in which a minute periscope is inserted through the abdominal wall. The most reliable method, however, is by serial ultrasound scans of the ovaries. Ovulation occurs 12–14 days before the onset of menstruation, so that it is correct to talk about ovulation at mid-cycle in one whose cycle averages 28 days, but in those who have a longer cycle, ovulation will occur after midcycle, as shown in Figure 24. In women with a 35-day cycle, ovulation is likely to occur about day 21, in those with a short cycle of 21 days it is more likely to occur about day 10.

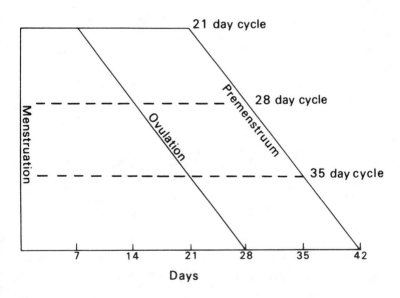

Figure 24   Timing of ovulation with different lengths of cycles

EMOTIONAL UPSET OF MENSTRUATION

The menstrual clock is a very delicate mechanism requiring an exact hormone balance to ensure a trouble-free menstruation. It is easily upset by stresses of all kinds, both happy events such as weddings, holidays and promotion, and unpleasant stresses like examinations, bereavements, and financial or marital problems.

The extent to which emotion can affect the timing of menstruation was shown in a study of 91 boarding school girls, who were all taking their tenth grade high school examinations in the second week of June. The average number menstruating each day before the examinations was 16 girls, but during the vital examination week as many as 36 girls were menstruating on one day. In fact, just under half showed an alteration in their normal menstrual pattern. In many the cycle was lengthened, in others it was shortened. In some, menstruation lasted longer, so that it spread over during examination week, but there were about a dozen girls who missed menstruation entirely that month. Clinical observation suggests that each individual's reaction to stress tends to remain the same throughout their menstruating years, so that the girls who missed menstruation at the time of examinations might also stop suddenly in later life if they were molested or their homes burnt down. Similarly, the others, who reacted with prolonged menstrual loss, might be expected to react in the same way under severe stress in later life.

One letter writer asked:

"Since my husband was killed in a sailing accident last year my periods have been very irregular and much heavier. I am now over the loss, have a new job, and only get depressed before a period. Is this anything to worry about?"

No, a horrible shock like that is bound to be felt by the hypothalamus, which in turn will temporarily upset the normal menstrual pattern. As the woman appears to be adjusting her life to the tragedy, it is likely that gradually her menstruation will return to its old pattern.

MENSTRUAL SYNCHRONY

Another point to be considered in relation to the timing of menstruation is what is called "menstrual synchrony," which is when a number of women's menstruations occur together. This happens among women who live close together in closed communities like communes, prisons, convents, college campuses and school dormitories; especially if they share common emotional experiences, such as examinations and end of term excitement, their menstruation gradually becomes synchronized. This in turn raises fresh problems, for it also means that if more than one woman is suffering from premenstrual tension, trouble is inevitable. Indeed, it may be necessary to move women prisoners from one cell to another before such synchronization occurs. Menstrual synchrony is frequently noticed in mothers and daughters. If a daughter is brought to the doctor by her mother and is unable to remember the date of her last menstruation, chances are that the mother will reply and then add, "our dates always come together." Similarly, menstruation tends to coincide in lesbians. The mechanism of this synchronization is not clear, but it has been suggested that it may be related to sensitive body odors.

The potency of these menstrual hormones is almost unbelievable. The powder a woman uses to cover the tip of her nose weighs many times more than the total amount of female hormones to be found in her blood stream. Yet they cause the sex organs and breasts to grow to mature size, and they bring about changes in bone structure and fat distribution which mold her figure into feminine contours and bring her to the peak of womanhood and motherhood.

SEX HORMONE BINDING GLOBULIN

Hormones are chemical messengers made in one organ and having their action on some other organ or tissue. Sex hormones can be attached, or bound, in the blood to a minute protein molecule called "globulin." The capacity of this sex hormone binding globulin (SHBG) to bind to dihydrotestosterone is measured in the SHBG blood test, mentioned in

Chapter 3 as a diagnostic aid for premenstrual syndrome. Just how this fits into the jigsaw of premenstrual syndrome is at present unknown. Why is the SHBG low in premenstrual syndrome? Why does the low SHBG rise when progesterone is administered to sufferers of premenstrual syndrome? Again, why does the SHBG fall when progestogens are administered? This only emphasizes the many riddles which are still awaiting solution in order to further our understanding of premenstrual syndrome.

HORMONE RECEPTORS

When a hormone has been conveyed in the blood to the tissue where its action is required, it is transported to the cell nucleus by means of a hormone receptor. Hormone receptors are situated within the tissue cells, and transport a single molecule of their special hormone through the cell wall, through the cell substance and the nuclear wall into the nucleus, where it is converted and used. Hormone receptors are very specific, and will only transport the special hormone for which they are made, be it thyroid, cortisone, estrogen or progesterone. There are no hormone receptors for the man-made progestogen drugs.

Progesterone receptors are present in the lining of the womb, where their presence is understandable, but the distribution of progesterone receptors in other parts of the body is of special interest. These tissues utilize progesterone in the luteal phases, although the precise function of the progesterone within these cells is not yet known. Progesterone receptors are widespread in the body, with the largest concentration found in the limbic area of the midbrain, a part that animal biologists refer to as the "area of rage and violence." It seems possible that it is an insufficiency of progesterone in the midbrain which is responsible for premenstrual tension. Progesterone receptors are also found in the nasopharangeal passages and lungs, and in the eyes, breasts and liver. This suggests that other premenstrual symptoms occur in just those areas known to have large numbers of progesterone receptors: the nasopharangeal passages and lungs, which are responsible for rhinitis, sinusitis, laryngitis and asthma;

the eyes, which are responsible for conjunctivitis, styes, uveitis and glaucoma; and the breasts, which are responsible for mastitis.

When progesterone is taken by mouth it passes via the portal system to the liver, the site of numerous progesterone receptors, where it is broken down and converted into other substances, which are different from the metabolic substances that result from the breakdown of progesterone in other tissues. With oral progesterone, therefore, the concentration of progesterone reaching the systemic blood is considerably lower.

With increasing knowledge has come the realization that hormones do not have a single action, but act on many systems. One has only to think of the widespread effects of an excess of thyroid, or a deficiency of insulin in diabetes. Thus, in addition to the action of estrogen on the reproductive system, estrogen is also involved in cholesterol balance, bone metabolism, blood circulation, and elasticity of the skin. Similarly, progesterone has other actions in the body, but they are not so well understood. It is certainly related to the regulation of blood sugar level, and the intracellular regulation of water, sodium and potassium, and probably also related to allergic reactions, cellular resistance to infection, and inflammatory reactions. Progesterone is also present in the adrenals in men, women and children, and is converted into other steroid hormones, such as cortisone, estrogen and testosterone.

16

What Goes Wrong?

THE PREMENSTRUAL SYNDROME

Apart from the recognition that premenstrual symptoms are eased by progesterone, there are many other factors which suggest that premenstrual syndrome is a progesterone responsive disease. For instance:

1) The symptoms are only present when progesterone should be present in the bloodstream, i.e., after ovulation up to menstruation. (Figure 25) The symptoms disappear when progesterone is absent from the bloodstream, i.e., after menstruation.

2) The onset is usually either at puberty, after a pregnancy, after taking the pill, or when menstruation returns after a long absence — all times of hormonal upset.

3) Symptoms are absent during pregnancy, when high amounts of progesterone are produced by the placenta.

4) Temperature charts confirm that the rise after ovulation may be poorly sustained in sufferers of the premenstrual syndrome. (See Victoria's temperature chart, Figure 26.)

5) The average progesterone level after ovulation is lower in sufferers of premenstrual syndrome than in normal women without menstrual symptoms. (Figure 27) Pro-

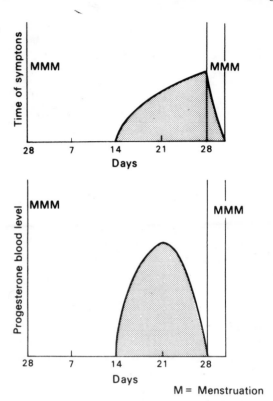

Figure 25 Timing of premenstrual syndrome and progesterone level during the menstrual cycle

fessor R. Taylor of the Premenstrual Clinic at St. Thomas's Hospital, London, found that out of 105 patients with premenstrual syndrome, roughly half had a lowered progesterone level in the second half of their cycle.

6) Premenstrual symptoms become worse when progestogens are administered, for progestogens are known to lower the blood progesterone level.

7) Symptoms start or increase in severity after sterilization, which is known to decrease the blood progesterone level.

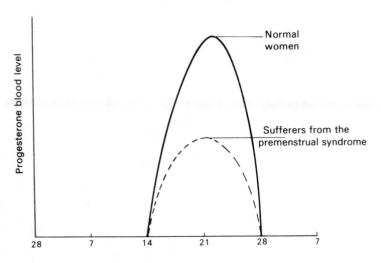

Figure 26   Progesterone in patients with the premenstrual syndrome and in normal women

8) Women with premenstrual syndrome have a low SHBG
   level, and progesterone raises the SHBG level in these
   women. The blood progesterone level is determined
   by radioimmunoassay, which can measure minute
   quantities of biological substances, but it must be
   remembered that progesterone is produced in spurts
   into the blood, and also that its level varies according
   to the particular day of the cycle and the presence of
   ovulation. This makes interpretation of progesterone
   levels difficult. Gynecologists measure the progesterone level on day 21 to determine whether a woman
   is ovulating, but premenstrual syndrome can occur
   whether or not a woman is ovulating.

Merely to say that there is a progesterone deficiency still
leaves many questions unanswered. For example:

a) Is there insufficient production of progesterone from
   the ovary?

b) Is there insufficient luteinising hormone (LH) produced by the pituitary gland?

c) Is there insufficient luteinising hormone releasing hormone (LHRH) produced by the hypothalamus?

d) Is the progesterone deficiency a true deficiency or does it appear so in comparison to the high estrogen levels so often found in sufferers of the syndrome?

e) Is the progesterone feedback pathway being blocked by too high a level of prolactin produced by the pituitary gland?

f) Is there a deficiency of sex hormone binding globulins, or in the mechanism needed to transport progesterone to the tissues?

g) Is there a deficiency of progesterone receptors in the tissue cells?

It is probable that individual cases of premenstrual syndrome fall into one or more of these groups, but up to now we have not been able to differentiate between these factors.

During pregnancy, considerably higher levels of progesterone are continuously present in the blood for nine months and not just present for two weeks and then absent for two weeks as in the non-pregnant woman. During the early weeks of pregnancy this extra progesterone is produced by the ovary, and as the placenta, or afterbirth, develops in the womb, it becomes a progesterone factory producing greater and greater amounts of progesterone. (Figure 27) During labor, after the baby is born, this placenta or progesterone factory comes away, and some women have difficulty in adjusting again to producing sufficient ovarian progesterone. It is these women who develop premenstrual syndrome and who often have pregnancies complicated by pre-eclampsia (high blood pressure and swelling of the ankles) or postnatal depression.

THE TIME OF ONSET

The onset of premenstrual syndrome is either at puberty, after a pregnancy, or after taking the pill. In those cases

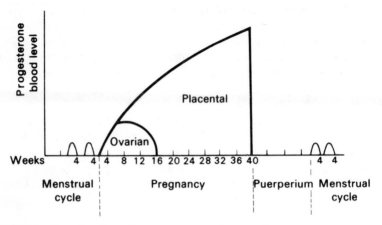

Figure 27   Levels of progesterone during the menstrual cycle and pregnancy

which start at puberty, the progesterone deficiency will have been present since the start of menstruation.

The pill contains a man-made artificial steroid called a "progestogen," which acts as a contraceptive and which also lowers the progesterone level in the blood (figure 34, p. 186). This means the pill produces a progesterone deficiency in those women whose progesterone production is not flexible enough to counteract the action of the progestogen.

The symptoms of premenstrual syndrome are many and various, but they all come under one or more of the following headings:

1) Water retention.

2) Lowered blood sugar.

3) Excess sodium and insufficient potassium at the cellular level.

4) Allergic reactions, e.g., asthma, rhinitis.

5) Lowered resistance to infection, e.g., boils, styes.

6) Inflammatory reactions, e.g., conjunctivitis.

It is possible that the symptoms related to water retention, lowered blood sugar, and altered sodium and potassium levels may be caused by a disturbance of the respective controlling centers in the hypothalamus. This is also a possible explanation for the last three groups of symptoms; alternatively, there may be an upset in the adrenal gland, for progesterone is also produced in the adrenals, where it is converted into the various adrenal hormones or corticosteroids. The corticosteroids have many functions, including that of mobilizing the mechanisms responsible for fighting infections and dealing with allergic reactions and inflammation.

From all this, it follows that the specific treatment for premenstrual syndrome is to make good the deficiency by administering progesterone. Information on progesterone treatment is given in Chapter 20.

FALL IN BLOOD SUGAR LEVEL

Progesterone also plays a part in the regulation of blood sugar (or blood glucose) level. To ensure that the blood sugar always remains close to the optimum level, we are provided with two regulating mechanisms, an upper and a lower. These prevent the blood sugar level from becoming too high (hyperglycemic), or too low (hypoglycemic), both of which may cause loss of consciousness or even death. (Figure 28) Essentially, the blood sugar level is maintained by eating carbohydrates, the energy-giving foods which include starches (flour, potatoes, oats, rye and rice), and sugars. The effect of eating sugars is to cause a rapid rise and rapid drop in blood sugar level, whereas ingestion of starches brings a more gradual and sustained rise. If we eat a large quantity of carbohydrates in one meal, the upper regulating mechanism is brought into play: there is a surge of insulin, and a valve opens, which releases the extra sugar into the urine (renal threshold). On the other hand, if there is a long interval without food and the blood sugar level drops too low, it may activate the lower regulating mechanism, causing a sudden outpouring of adrenalin. This adrenalin mobilizes some of the sugar stored in other cells of the body and passes it into the blood, so that the blood sugar level is again restored to the optimum level.

(Figure 28) However, when sugar is taken from the cells, they fill up with water, and this is responsible for water retention, bloatedness, and weight gain.

When a woman takes some food, such as a breakfast of eggs and toast, the blood sugar level rises immediately and then falls gradually over the next four hours. If she takes some more food after three or four hours, the blood sugar will again rise immediately and then fall slowly. However, if she does not take any food for a long interval, the blood sugar will continue to drop until it reaches the lower regulating mechanism, or baseline.

Progesterone is involved in the lower regulating mechanism and if, before menstruation, there is insufficient progesterone, the baseline is raised. (Figure 29) This means that women with premenstrual syndrome will tend to reach the level at which the lower regulating mechanism comes into action at an earlier stage; in practice it is usually about three hours after the ingestion of starchy food, so women are

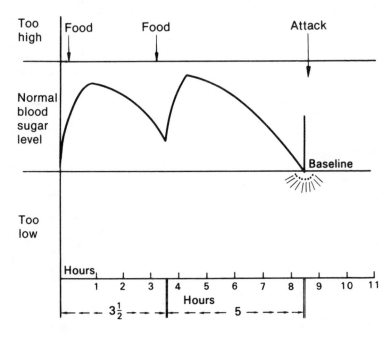

Figure 28   Effect of food on blood sugar levels

advised to ensure that they eat small portions of starchy food every three hours. Men, on the other hand, can usually go longer without replenishment, as their lower regulating mechanism is set at a different level.

These attacks, brought on by fasting and a resulting drop in blood sugar level, are sometimes erroneously called "hypoglycemic attacks"; doctors do not like that usage as the term "hypoglycemic" is reserved for those whose blood sugar stays below the baseline and below the normal blood sugar level. In the case of normal women, Nature's fail-safe control prevents hypoglycemia from occurring.

Adrenalin is the hormone which also mobilizes the body's responses for "fright, fight and flight," and a sudden outpouring of adrenalin may be enough to trigger fits of irritability, migraine, panic, or epilepsy. In others, it might cause feelings of being weak, shivery and faint, or bring on palpitations. On the other hand, there are also those fortunate individuals who can manage long fasts, as they are unaware when their

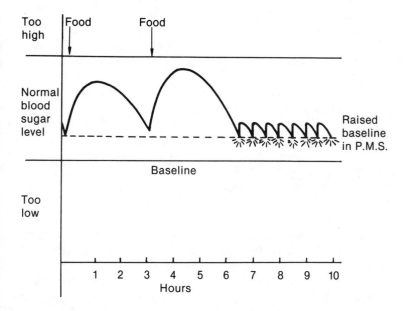

Figure 29 Effect of food on blood sugar levels in women with premenstrual syndrome

blood sugar baseline has been reached, and they get renewed energy from their own sugar stores.

Many women will have noticed that they can easily diet and go five hours without food after menstruation, but they have marked food cravings before menstruation. Giving progesterone helps to correct this premenstrual alteration of the blood sugar level.

SPASMODIC DYSMENORRHEA

It has already been mentioned that spasmodic dysmenorrhea is the opposite of premenstrual syndrome, and there are several factors which suggest that an estrogen deficiency is the cause of these period pains. For instance:

1) It does not start with the first menstruation, but only when ovulation occurs.

2) It is relieved by a full-term pregnancy.

3) If a pregnancy does not intervene, a gradual reduction in pain after the age of 25 years is usual.

4) The pain is relieved by the pill or estrogen administration.

5) The sufferers tend to be immature, with poor breast development and sparse hair in their armpits.

6) It is frequently accompanied by acne.

In puberty, estrogen is responsible for the development of the secondary sex characteristics. It is responsible for pubertal breast development, for the growth of hair in the armpits and lower abdomen, for the development and enlargement of the womb, and more especially for developing the muscles of the womb and ensuring it has a good blood supply. Estrogen also decreases the production of grease in the skin and so prevents acne, and is also involved in the reduction of prostaglandin releases during menstruation.

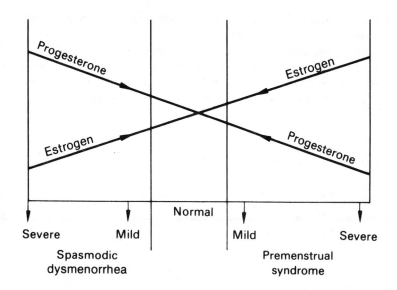

Figure 30 Arbitrary levels of progesterone and estrogen

If ovular menstruation occurs before the womb is fully developed, the door to the womb is not supple enough to open easily for the flow of menstrual blood. It is rather like trying to blow up a balloon for the first time, which is very difficult. But if it has once been fully inflated, then on the next occasion it is easy to inflate. If the womb is gradually stretched during the nine months of pregnancy, then subsequently the door will open up at menstruation without pain. Or, if the muscles of the womb are gradually extended by the prolonged action of estrogen, the painful periods are gradually eased during the mid-twenties.

TWO HORMONAL TYPES

Thus, it would seem that the two common period problems, premenstrual syndrome and spasmodic dysmenorrhea, are related to a deficiency in the levels of the two menstrual hormones — progesterone and estrogen, respectively. Figure 30 is a diagram of the effect of these two hormone levels on an individual. A marked progesterone deficiency will cause severe premenstrual syndrome. On the other hand, a moderately low estrogen level will only cause mild spasmodic dysmenorrhea, but a severe estrogen deficiency will cause severe period pains. In between these extremes are those fortunate women who do not experience any problems with menstruation. Although women may move slightly up and down this scale during the course of their lives, the movement will tend to stay within the limits of the same group, unless either progesterone or estrogen is given or a pregnancy occurs. These two groups of women tend to have other common characteristics, which are discussed below.

PROGESTERONE DEFICIENT GROUP

Women in the premenstrual syndrome group will tend to be fertile, but their pregnancies may be followed by postnatal depression, and they are more prone to depressive illnesses and high blood pressure during their life span. Among those who become pregnant, one in every five will be likely to have pre-eclamptic toxemia, with a marked gain in weight and high blood pressure during pregnancy, while the others will blossom in pregnancy, being free from their usual premenstrual migraine, asthma and depression, and will later look back on the last months of pregnancy as the healthiest days of their life. These women, if given estrogen, will tend to get side effects, as they already have a high level of this hormone. They will be prone to minor side effects like nausea, gain in weight, headaches and depression, but will also risk more serious ones, like thrombosis. The pill contains estrogen together with a synthetic progestogen, and as already mentioned, progestogens lower the normal progesterone level in the blood, making their existing progesterone deficiency worse.

ESTROGEN DEFICIENT GROUP

On the other hand, women with spasmodic dysmenorrhea will grow out of their period pains, either following pregnancy or during their mid-twenties, and thereafter will have trouble-free menstruations. These are the women who feel positively better on the pill, even preferring the ones with a relatively higher dose of estrogen as these boost their low estrogen levels. However, at the menopause their already low estrogen levels are not helped by the declining estrogen output from the ovaries, so these women are likely to develop menopausal symptoms early, even before menstruation has stopped. Unless they are given estrogen replacement treatment during the menopausal years, they are likely to be the ones who suffer most from the ending of their childbearing years.

As with other hormonal disorders, it is not surprising to find that there is a marked family tendency, with daughters, sisters and mothers belonging to the same menstrual hormonal group — either progesterone deficient or estrogen deficient. Studies in twins have suggested that, among identical twins, if one suffers from premenstrual syndrome then the other will too, whereas in unidentical twins, the incidence of premenstrual syndrome is the same as that found among sisters. Similarly, adopted daughters are likely to take the pattern of their natural mother in respect to either premenstrual syndrome or spasmodic dysmenorrhea, and not the pattern of their adopted mother.

MISSED PERIODS

> "Married hopes and unmarried fear
> Are the common causes of amenorrhea"

Amenorrhea is the absence of periods, and the above quoted nurses' jingle is a reminder that the most common cause of a missed menstruation is pregnancy. Often, if the girl is single, it is more likely to be a delayed period. If she normally has a long cycle of perhaps 33–36 days, has not kept a record of her cycles, and has run a risk during the month, she is likely to be fearful on every day after the 28th day that she might be pregnant. Unfortunately, the routine pregnancy test cannot be used reliably until two weeks after the missed period, or 42 days since the last period, and this is an awfully long time to wait. However, there would usually be the tell-tale signs of an early pregnancy, such as morning sickness, getting up to urinate at night, and painful enlarging breasts. A blood test can recognize a pregnancy within seven days of conception, which is even before the missed period, and serial ultrasound scans of the ovaries will also detect an early pregnancy. However, both of these methods are expensive and are not universally available. There was a hormonal pregnancy test in which estrogen and progestogen tablets were taken and, if the woman was not pregnant, vaginal bleeding would occur within 48 hours. This test has now been stopped because there is an ever-present risk that, should the woman be pregnant, there might be fetal abnormalities.

Missed periods may occur quite normally at puberty, during the first three years after the onset of menstruation, during breastfeeding, and again at the menopause. In the last case, menstruation has often started to get shorter and the loss lighter before a period is actually missed.

To find the other causes of missed menstruation one must return to the hormonal controlling system, for any upset to the hormonal pathway may disturb the normal rhythm of menstruation. Stress is perhaps the most common cause:

> A friend, *Winifred*, with two children, had been visiting us, but when she returned to her home she found a fire engine outside and her house aflame. She stopped menstruating for eleven weeks.

Nor is it necessary for the stress to be so unpleasant; it can just as easily happen following happy circumstances.

> *Yvonne*, a 25-year-old graphic artist, had a wonderful romance on a Greek island and stopped menstruating for nine weeks after she returned.

In both these cases it was the result of messages from the brain affecting the menstrual clock, situated in the hypothalamus.

Factors which disturb the other controlling centers in the hypothalamus (see Figure 21) will also upset the menstrual clock. Common among these are rapid weight changes, especially anorexia nervosa or even rigid dieting which does not quite reach the proportions of anorexia nervosa. Each woman has her own critical weight level, and if her weight falls below this level then menstruation will stop and will not return until her weight reaches the critical level. Therefore, those with a tendency to weight loss and missed menstruation are advised to weigh themselves each time menstruation occurs, so as to learn their own personal weight limits. Depressive illnesses may also delay menstruation, and again, it is unlikely for the periods to return naturally until the depression is a thing of the past. Other chronic systemic illnesses such as tuberculosis and acute rheumatic fever may halt menstruation temporarily.

Lack of menstruation after stopping the pill is an example of the ovary having been prevented from ovulating for so long that the menstrual clock has also been halted; and even when the pill is discontinued, the menstrual clock does not restart automatically. Often, when it does restart after a long interval, the cycles are found to be anovular. This indicates that ovulation has not restarted, although menstruation has, and pregnancy is therefore impossible. Fortunately, nowadays this can be corrected by appropriate hormone treatment.

TOO MUCH

Another problem is when menstruation goes on for too long, comes too often, or is too heavy — in short, when there is too much of it. Again, stress can be the cause, although never in those women who on other occasions miss their menstruation at times of stress.

> *Zena,* a 45-year-old wife of a T.V. producer, bled for nine weeks continuously, starting on the day her dream house, on which she had already put a deposit, was sold to a higher bidder without her knowledge.

There is an interesting example in Mark's Gospel:

> "And there was a woman who had a flow of blood for twelve years, and who had suffered much under many physicians, and had spent all that she had, and was no

better, but rather grew worse. She had heard the reports about Jesus, and came up behind him in the crowd and touched his garment. For she said, 'If I touch even his garments, I shall be made well.' And immediately the hemorrhage ceased, and she felt in her body that she was healed of her disease." (5, 25–29, RSV)

This incident can be seen in the light of our present medical knowledge. This woman had faith, and the tremendous emotional release of being able actually to go up and touch the clothes that Jesus was wearing was sufficient stimulus to her menstrual clock to correct her prolonged menstruation.

Hormone therapy when taking the pill, and more especially the progestogen-only pill, may cause prolonged breakthrough bleeding, which can be a great nuisance and is a sign that treatment needs adjusting.

Occasionally, there may be bleeding at ovulation; this is usually lighter and only lasts from an hour or two to one or two days, but if there is no regular record of the bleeding, it may not be easily recognized. A menstrual chart will clearly show the difference between the regular mid-cycle bleeding, which is harmless, and the totally irregular bleeding which needs gynecological investigation.

Conditions which increase the surface area of the lining of the womb will result in heavy or prolonged bleeding. Examples are polyps, or fibroids, which are situated near the cavity of the womb. However, as there is always the chance that the extra bleeding may be the result of a malignant condition, there is always justification in asking for a full examination.

Occasionally, an intra-uterine device (IUD), whether a coil, loop, or copper seven, may cause excessive bleeding or prolonged scanty bleeding for several days before and after menstruation. Although hormone treatment may be tried to stop the excessive bleeding, it is often best to remove the device and reinsert another in a more comfortable position. Sometimes a device has been in for years without any trouble, and then gradually menstruation gets more prolonged. This is usually a sign that the device is starting to dislodge and may indeed be pushed out of the womb and into the vagina.

Sometimes, bleeding which is thought to be menstrual is caused by the bleeding of an ulcer, or erosion, at the cervix or opening of the womb. This can easily be spotted by a doctor on examination, and he may well cauterize it.

17

The Vacant Plot

Can anyone blame the woman who for years has endured wretched miseries each month, if she dreams of the day when those troublesome organs will be removed by one clean swoop of the surgeon's knife? Already it is such a commonplace procedure that it is known as the "Birthday Operation," to be celebrated during the 40th year. Today, the operative risks associated with the removal of the womb are minimal, but is it really the answer to a woman's prayers?

It is no good asking the gynecologist, for he sees the woman a few months later, examines the scar to ensure it's well-healed, assures her that she'll never again menstruate, possibly prescribes some estrogen tablets, and says goodbye. It is better to ask the family doctor, who will care for this woman, not just for one year, but for the next twenty.

There are many very good reasons for the removal of the womb, and possibly the ovaries as well. At the top of that list would come the possibility of any malignancy, and no doctor will disagree here. Sometimes it is performed because of fibroids — when they are either so large that they are interfering with some other organ, or so numerous that they are causing heavy menstruation — or because of endometriosis, and again these cases are certainly justified. At the other end of the scale, there are those women who demand it so as to be 100% contraceptively safe, probably feeling that they cannot take even the very small risk that goes with the pill or a device, or possibly having already tried these methods without success. A 42-year-old owner of a boutique confessed that she changed her gynecologist seven times before she found one who was prepared to remove her womb for contraception. She stated that she was not convinced that sterilization would be reliable enough.

Far too many women have the operation in order to overcome their premenstrual syndrome. They would be better advised to have this condition treated with progesterone therapy. No one will disagree that on many occasions the symptoms are so severe that drastic treatment is warranted; unfortunately, a hysterectomy is not the answer. One well-known gynecologist who diagnoses premenstrual syndrome explains to the woman that this is due to progesterone deficiency, does a hysterectomy, and then refers her to the Premenstrual Syndrome Clinic for progesterone treatment.

Many of the problems for which the operation is recommended could be treated much more successfully with hormone therapy.

The immediate post-operative weeks are usually pleasant and uneventful, but whether the womb only or the womb plus the ovaries are removed, there is still an irreparable break in the hormonal pathway, (Figure 22) and the menstrual clock, which is not touched by the operation, receives a severe jolt. Within 6–8 days there is an increase in follicle stimulating hormone (FSH) from the pituitary, and within 8–10 days an increase in luteinising hormone (LH). The menstrual clock starts reacting to the lack of information from the womb, and within a further three weeks there is a threefold increase in follicle stimulating hormone and a two-fold increase in luteinising hormone. This occurs whether or not the ovaries have been removed, although the increase is not so great if an estrogen implant is given at the time of operation.

The changes which occur with the surgical removal of the womb or ovaries are known as an "artificial" menopause, and should not be confused with the natural menopause. In a natural menopause the estrogen is given continuously, as there is no risk of estrogen causing a build up of the lining of the womb. If the depression is cyclical, it will respond to progesterone. Again, progesterone should be given continuously, even if ovulation is occurring, for there is no longer the possibility of causing irregularity of menstruation. The changes in natural menopause occur gradually over several years, with a slow closing down of the menstrual clock and shrinking of the ovaries and womb; in an artificial menopause the changes are sudden, and only affect the womb and/or the ovaries, leaving the menstrual clock intact.

All goes well after the operation for some 6–12 months, but then the hormonal difference between the two groups of women discussed on page 140 begins to show itself. Those who previously suffered from premenstrual syndrome will find that the usual cyclical symptoms return. The husband is often the first to notice it, and he will try to remind his wife of what is happening. Or she may recognize the telltale headache, which previously ushered in a period, and which now assumes the proportions of a prostrating migraine.

> *Angela*, the 48-year-old wife of a USAF colonel, had a successful hysterectomy for fibroids which were causing heavy bleeding. She made an excellent recovery and assumed full household duties until nine months later, when she suddenly had four days of extreme tiredness. She stayed in bed, attributing it to 'flu or some nasty virus. The following month it recurred, but this time she stayed in bed for six days. Gradually the duration of the tiredness lengthened until it represented two weeks in each month. It would start gradually with mere tiredness, and she would manage to keep up for a few days, but then bed became essential. The end of the attacks was quite definite, and afterwards she had no other symptoms and resumed her normal social life.
>
> Her husband had kept a meticulous diary, from which a chart was constructed. When first seen, she had already had nine months of this distressing condition, which fortunately responded completely to progesterone treatment.

Invariably premenstrual syndrome is more marked after a hysterectomy than before, and there may also be extra symptoms.

> One woman, a part-time worker, was first seen after she had been charged at the police station. Two years previously a hysterectomy had been carried out. Prior to the operation she had suffered from premenstrual tension and headaches.

After the operation her premenstrual syndrome had increased in severity, and for a few days each month she would also experience breast fullness and a distressing feeling of unreality and confusion. She related these episodes to the time of her expected premenstruum and carefully charted the days on a calendar. She even went so far as to arrange her work schedule so as to avoid these inevitable confused days. In Court she described these days of confusion, explaining that sometimes she would come home having bought items she did not need, such as dog food when she had no dogs, curry and other foods which she never ate, and underwear which was the wrong size. She was in a daze and could not recall what had happened. The day of her offense had been such a day. Even when she was taken to the police station by a plain-clothes policeman after having been charged, she thought the officer was a rapist driving down an unknown road. The case was dismissed. She has since been under progesterone treatment, and is now free from cyclical confusion and premenstrual syndrome.

While carrying out a nationwide survey into the hormonal factors of migraine in women in 1975, it was noted that it was those women with a history of premenstrual syndrome who stated that the severity of their migraine had been increased by a hysterectomy. Their three-month charts, giving the precise timing of migraine attacks, confirmed that the attacks were still occurring cyclically.

One cannot emphasize too strongly the need for women with cyclical symptoms to keep a careful record of their problem days, even if they have had their womb or ovaries removed. Sometimes, when women feel very depressed and are unable to record their days of depression because the onset is so gradual, it is just as useful for them to record the days on which they have breast symptoms, as these are usually very definite and commonplace. Alternatively, they can just record the days when they are feeling really well with a [✓].

Brenda, a 47-year-old, began her consultation with a detailed account of how her husband had been moved from one town to another, and how she had made a suicide attempt within days of their move and had been hospitalized for several months. Within a week or two of her discharge she moved back to her previous home, but made another suicide attempt the following week and was again admitted. It was only after taking a long and confused history, assisted by her husband, that discovery was made of a hysterectomy and the fact that she was now experiencing cyclical attacks of depression and moodiness. Once the cyclical nature of her symptoms was appreciated and confirmed by a two-month record, it was possible to give her progesterone treatment and restore her to normality.

Two recent surveys have emphasized the high incidence of depression occurring in women one to three years after a hysterectomy, with or without the removal of the ovaries. The depression appears to be greatest in those under 40 years at the time of the operation; those with a previous history of depression, especially postnatal depression; those in whom no gynecological abnormality could be found by the pathologist who examined the womb after operation (in one of the surveys, 45% of the wombs were reported to be normal); and in those women who had a history of marital disruption.

Dr. Ronald Richards, a general practitioner in Oxford, England, observed that patients who had previously undergone a hysterectomy often had medical notes bulging out of their files, so that at a glance one realized that they had already done the rounds of most hospital departments. His survey, confirmed by others, emphasized the high incidence of depression in those with a history of a hysterectomy.

My paper on "The Aftermath of Hysterectomy," read at the Royal Society of Medicine in London in 1957, revealed that 44% of women had either been divorced, separated, or had sought the assistance of a marriage guidance counselor since the operation. A husband is more likely to be sympathetic when a woman is ill each month with menstrual problems than he is when, after the operation, she flies into rages for no apparent reason. One husband said, "She used to have a reason for it, but now she's quite unpredictable";

and another, "I had hoped the operation would make her more even-tempered."

Another disturbing finding in the survey was that more than half the women gained more than 28 lbs. in weight in the year following their hysterectomy. How often is a woman warned before the operation that the odds are two to one that such a marked weight-gain might occur? The reason for the depression and weight-gain after hysterectomy may be appreciated by recognizing the proximity of the menstrual clock to the mood controlling center and the weight controlling center in the hypothalamus. (Figure 21)

There would seem to be two types of post-hysterectomy depression: a cyclical depression, and a continuous depression. The continuous depression is likely to be suffered by those who experienced spasmodic dysmenorrhea in their youth, and have a tendency to be estrogen deficient. These women respond very well to estrogen therapy, which needs to be continued not only through their depressive illness, but even after the time of the natural menopause.

A few women are found to have a high prolactin level, suggesting that the operation has caused a disturbance in the hypothalamic-pituitary mechanism. These women respond well to bromocriptine, a drug which lowers the prolactin level.

In theory, the removal of the womb should have no effect on subsequent sexual activity. The vagina and clitoris are untouched at operation and, if anything, sexual activity should be enhanced once the fear of a possible pregnancy is permanently removed. In practice, however, there are those who previously had a satisfactory sex life who now suddenly find they have lost all urge and satisfaction. If this occurs, it is well worth seeking professional help; often testosterone is the magic restorative.

Perhaps it is relevant to mention that when apes have had their wombs removed, their partner also rejects them; but if the ape has only been given a mock operation, without the womb being removed, the couple enjoy a natural sexual relationship. Whether a similar effect occurs in humans is not yet known; one can only guess.

18

Menopausal Miseries

It is only children who long to grow old — adults hate the very thought of it. This is never more true than when the menopause approaches, for many see this as a door leading to senility, when it is really the gateway to an era of serenity; an era characterized by confidence, calmness, sophistication, stable moods, and endless energy.

Women are unique in the animal kingdom as the only females who outlive their reproductive function and can then enjoy up to half their lifespan without it. The end of menstruation occurs according to an individual pre-arranged plan. The menstrual clock runs at its own individual rate; in some it runs on a little longer, in others it stops earlier.

The word "menopause" means the pausing of menstruation, and more precisely, the last menstruation. It is the reverse of the menarche, but it cannot be timed as accurately because it is only seen in retrospect; only when there have been no further menstruations for a year can it be dated exactly. Earlier, the term "climacteric" was used to cover the years before and after the last menstruation, a time when the changes in the reproductive system were occurring. Nowadays it is usual to use the term "menopause" more loosely to cover those years of hormonal change.

HORMONAL CHANGES

As with all the changes Nature makes in our reproductive system, those at the menopause are very gradual, taking 5–7 years to complete. First, there is the gradual missing of ovulation. Studies in which small sections of the normal lining of

152

the womb have been removed and examined microscopically have suggested that the occasional anovular cycle can occur up to six years before the last menstruation. Gradually, missed ovulations become more frequent, and the menstrual flow may become lighter and scanty. As the ovary declines, the hypothalamus and pituitary try to stimulate it with an increased output of the two hormones, follicle stimulating hormone (FSH) and luteinising hormone (LH). But the ovaries are unable to respond, and their production of estrogen and progesterone gradually decreases until, some years later, it comes to an end. Thus the presence of the menopause can be determined by blood tests showing a low level of estradiol and a raised level of FSH.

It has already been stated that the main functions of estrogen are the rebuilding of the lining of the womb after it has been shed at menstruation, the alteration of the cervical mucus to assist fertilization, and breast development. It also has some other functions, which are of importance after the menstruating years are finished. Estrogen promotes the cholesterol balance, nourishes the blood circulatory system, increases the elasticity of the skin, and is involved in the building up of bones. Throughout life, the adrenal glands in men and women build up progesterone from cholesterol and then convert the progesterone further into estrogen, testosterone, cortisone and other steroids. When estrogen is no longer produced by the ovaries, it continues to be produced in the adrenal glands, which have always produced a small amount, and in the peripheral tissues. After menopause it is this non-ovarian estrogen which has to fulfill the other functions for the blood, bones and skin. All too often there is insufficient estrogen for these other tasks, either temporarily during the changeover time or permanently, and it is this lack of estrogen which is responsible for all the unpleasant symptoms of the menopause. Then the woman, once her ovaries decline, is left to carry on with an insufficiency of this vital and powerful female hormone.

Up to the age of 40 years, narrowing of the arteries — and particularly narrowing of the blood vessels of the heart — is between 10 and 40 times more common in men than in women. After the menopause, as the circulating estrogen decreases, there is a marked increase in this incidence in women, so that gradually the differences between men and women become less. But it is not until the age of 75 years that the incidence is equal. After a hysterectomy, the incidence of narrowing of the arteries and of the coronary vessels is increased fourfold as compared with premenopausal women. Also, among those few women who have a premature menopause before the age of 40 years, there is a sevenfold increase in coronary thrombosis. So the presence of estrogen in the blood is very important in preventing narrowing of the arteries and the occurrence of coronary disease.

Bones are not stable, unchanging structures. Throughout life, new bone cells are being laid down and old ones removed. This needs calcium, phosphorus, vitamins and other minerals, and also estrogen. This is why everyone, men, women and children included, has a small amount of estrogen circulating in the blood. This estrogen is produced by the two adrenal glands. After the menopause some women, who have relied during their menstruating life on the estrogen produced by the ovaries, may find they have insufficient estrogen being made by the adrenals, and this leads to thinning of the bones. This thinning of the bones shows up on X-rays, and ten years after the menopause it is present in 40% of all women. Although this can be halted with estrogen administration, it takes another ten years before the X-rays show any improvement.

Progesterone is no longer required to prepare the lining of the womb or the cervical mucus for possible pregnancy after menstruation ceases, but progesterone also has another function. All through life, in both sexes, progesterone is built up in the adrenal glands from cholesterol, and immediately converted into estrogen, testosterone, cortisone and the other adrenal hormones, or corticosteriods, which have various jobs to do throughout the body. As ovarian progesterone is only present in the blood stream for half of each cycle, the adrenals generally manage to make enough for their own needs during the menstruating years, and so they are usually capable of carrying on this task after the menopause. This is why progesterone deficiency is no longer a problem after the menopause, although if progesterone is given it can be converted into estrogen.

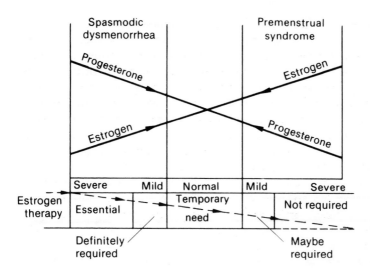

Figure 31 Need for estrogen therapy at the menopause

TWO HORMONAL GROUPS

Earlier, in Chapter 16, the two hormonal types, the estrogen deficient and progesterone deficient, were discussed. But apart from spasmodic dysmenorrhea, most of the previous chapters have dealt with the progesterone deficient group, and the havoc that can be caused by premenstrual syndrome in the home, at work and at leisure. At the menopause we again turn our attention to the estrogen deficient group, for these are the women whose menopausal sufferings begin earliest and are the most severe. This can be seen in Figure 31, which shows that those women who had spasmodic dysmenorrhea in their teens and then sufficient estrogen for normal menstruation nevertheless suffer most from menopausal symptoms; indeed, the chances are that they will experience menopausal symptoms while their menstruation is still regularly occurring each month. Their need for estrogen therapy at the menopause is essential, and they are the ones who will probably need it for many years to come. Those who were in the normal category may require estrogen therapy during the

156   ONCE A MONTH

changeover period, but will probably manage to make enough
for their own requirements thereafter. The sufferers of mild
premenstrual syndrome may require estrogen temporarily when
their menstruations first stop, but should gradually manage
without. On the other hand, the severe premenstrual syndrome sufferers are those who will probably have no need for
estrogen, either during the menopausal years or later; these
women have always managed to have a high estrogen level by
supplementing the ovarian estrogen with that which is produced in the adrenals.

In short, it is a case of roundabouts and swings. Those
who had greatest difficulties with premenstrual monthly problems can look forward to a problem-free era, while those
who had little trouble during the twenties and thirties are the
ones with most problems at the menopause.

It will be noted that the term "Hormone Replacement
Treatment," or HRT, has not been used because this only
leads to confusion, for both estrogen and progesterone are
hormones and both are used in replacement therapy.

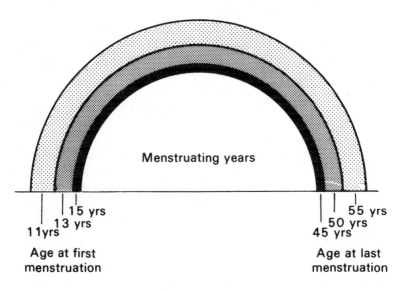

Figure 32   Relation between the age of menarche
and menopause

AGE OF MENOPAUSE

In the United States, the average age of the menopause is 52 years, while in Britain it is 48 years, with a range between 45 and 55 years. Those whose menstruation ceases before 45 years are said to have a "premature menopause".

The exact time of the menopause is very individual. However, a study of the following four factors can give some indication as to whether it will be early or late:

1) The age of menarche. The effect of this is that those who start menstruation early tend to finish late, giving a "rainbow" effect, as shown in Figure 32.

2) The hormonal group. Those in the estrogen deficient group have a tendency to finish menstruation before the average, while sufferers from premenstrual syndrome tend to finish after 50 years of age.

3) Genetic factors. Some families give a story of the mother, sister and aunts all finishing menstruation early, in which case such a patient may also expect to finish early. For this reason, it is worth finding out what age the mother had her last normal menstruation.

4) Smoking. A survey at the BUPA Medical Center in London showed that at 48–49 years, 36% of smokers were post-menopausal compared with 23% non-smokers; four years later, the figures were 89% smokers and 71% non-smokers. So smoking habits should also be considered when estimating the probable age at which the menopause may occur.

PATTERNS OF ENDING

Among those women who regularly record the dates of their menstruation, it may be observed that the menstruating years end in a wide variety of ways. Three patterns are recognizable, but even then, some women may find that their own individual ending covers more than one pattern:

a) There may be a gradual ending, so that whereas menstruation initially lasted four or five days, it gradually lasts one or two days, then only one day or even one hour monthly. Nevertheless, the cycle is maintained and menstruation comes when expected.

b) There may be the occasional missed menstruation, possibly just an odd one, and then menstruation resumes again for a month or two before another is missed. Gradually, there are more missed menstruations than actual menstruations, but each menstruation lasts the expected number of days, say four to six days.

c) There is a sudden ending of menstruation, which had previously been regular, with the final menstruation lasting the normal or nearly normal number of days. This abrupt ending is most likely to coincide with a stressful event, such as a daughter's wedding, moving, or becoming a grandparent. This abrupt ending may even be the start of a depressive illness.

The individual woman's attitude to a missed or delayed menstruation depends upon her recent sexual activity and desire for pregnancy. If there has been no sexual activity, she may not notice the infrequency or absence of menstrual bleeding for a month or two; but if the possibility of pregnancy exists, her attitude changes to one of concern, with increasing happiness or unhappiness as each additional day of missed menstruation confirms the diagnosis. The possibility of pregnancy is usually uppermost in the minds of those whose regular menstruation suddenly ceases, and it is the most common cause in the earlier years. After 45 years of age, however, one must always first consider the possibility that menopause has begun. Comments by patients in this predicament include:

"I don't want to get my name in the *Guiness Book of Records* as the oldest Mother in the world."

"I would hate to be drawing my old age pension when my child is at school."

And from a grandmother:

"My child would then be younger than her niece."

Usually it is quite easy for a doctor to tell if a patient is pregnant or undergoing the menopause. If she is pregnant, her breasts will be full, she may have symptoms of morning sickness and of passing urine during the night, and on examination her vagina is moist and the neck of the womb soft. On the other hand, if she is entering her menopause, her breasts will begin to decrease in size, she may have menopausal symptoms, especially hot flushes, and on examination her vagina will be pale and dry and the neck of the womb firm and smaller.

MENOPAUSAL FLUSHES

The most characteristic symptom of the menopause is the "hot flush," or "flash." It is a sensation of burning heat, arising from the waist and passing up to the top of the head. It only lasts a few minutes, five minutes at the most, and may be either visible, when the skin becomes flushed and beads of sweat appear, or invisible. Very few women, indeed, pass through the menopausal years without experiencing a single flush, which may range in frequency from only one or two a week to between fifty and a hundred a day. Many women are embarrassed by them, but others working with women of their own age can laugh about them, believing that "a flush shared is a flush halved." Our grandparents used to say they were worth "a dollar a flush." They may be accompanied by palpitations, fluttering in the chest, or a feeling of choking, apprehension or anxiety. Flushes are worse immediately after a hot drink or spicy foods.

The flushes can occur at night, when the woman usually awakens abruptly in a bath of sweat; these are known as "night sweats." When the wife suddenly flings off the bedclothes, the husband is more likely to be annoyed rather than sympathetic.

A story is told about a group of women undergraduates at Girton College, Cambridge, in the 20s, who were discussing the menopausal problems and hot flushes that were being experienced by their mothers and counselors. They agreed that as they were all so emancipated and fully understood the facts of life, they would never have to suffer the ordeal of flushes. They formed a Menopause Club, promising to keep in touch with each other and give full accounts of how they fared through that great age. When the time came, each one of them experienced the flushes and other menopausal symptoms to a greater or lesser extent, in spite of their full knowledge of the events of life.

It would appear that the flushes are due to a sudden stimulus to the temperature controlling center in the hypothalamus, and are associated with a rise in the follicle stimulating hormone and luteinising hormone from the pituitary, as well as a deficiency of estrogen.

MENOPAUSAL SYMPTOMS

The symptoms are usually divided into two groups: specific symptoms, which are caused by estrogen deficiency and can be relieved by giving estrogen, and the vague psychological symptoms, some of which may be relieved by estrogen and some not, depending on the individual patient. Non-specific symptoms include tiredness, insomnia, irritability, depression, headaches, palpitations, anxiety, dizziness, forgetfulness and absentmindedness.

Lack of estrogen may cause the vagina to become dry, pale and thin, which in turn may cause itching, pain or frequency in passing urine (often misdiagnosed as cystitis), pain on initial penetration at intercourse and ultimately, loss of sex drive.

The skin becomes paler and thinner, and loses its elasticity so that wrinkles develop, especially on the face around the eyes and mouth and in the neck. The soaring sales of cosmetics and beauty treatments, and the demand for cosmetic surgery, are evidence of the obvious distress caused by these middle age symptoms.

The rheumatic-like pains that develop in the bones, muscles and joints are due to the thinning of the bones. There is often marked stiffness on rising in the mornings, and the pains tend to move about from one site to another over the course of weeks. Sometimes the joints of the fingers may become very painful, with marked swelling, and then as the pain and swelling ease the joint may be left deformed and misaligned. In the postmenopausal years, fractures of the wrist, neck of the femur, and crushed fractures of the spine are a sign of marked thinning of the bones. The "dowager's hump" at the top of the spine is also a sign of thinning of the bones, but this does not develop until the seventies.

The thinning of the bones also causes a decrease in body height. Leonardo da Vinci, in his "Universal Man," demonstrated that the height equals the armspan, and so it is for men and premenopausal women. However, as a woman's vertebrae become thinner after the menopause there is a decrease in height, with no corresponding decrease in armspan. If there is more than an inch and a half loss of height compared with armspan, it is an indication that the woman should be on long-term estrogen therapy. (Figure 33)

The worst symptoms are the non-specific ones, which led to the following comments:

"I think I must be going insane."

"I feel so harassed; the whole world seems to be resting on my shoulders."

"It's even tougher than pregnancy and labor."

At the menopause there are mood changes which are continuous, not mood swings which last only two weeks or so at a time and are then eased, temporarily at least. It may turn an easy-going type into a shrew, a highly-strung individual into a crying hysteric, a happy-go-lucky woman into a restless, nagging bundle of nerves, and a placid housewife into an absent-minded professor who puts the cat in the refrigerator and the milk on the doorstep. At this time, many women leave the femininity rat-race, and their personality factors become more important and possibly exaggerated. Even the woman's shape alters as her breasts begin to sag, and she develops middle-aged spread. There is a tendency for the thin to become even thinner and the fat to become obese.

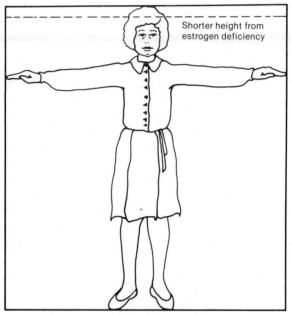

Normally the armspan equals the height, but if estrogen deficiency occurs at the menopause the armspan exceeds the height

Figure 33 Relation between armspan and height

DIAGNOSIS

The diagnosis is usually not difficult to make on clinical grounds. The hot flushes are most characteristic, but it must not be forgotten that some anti-depressants can also cause flushes. The thin skin, the greying hair, the wrinkles, the dry vagina and deformed fingers and toes are all telltale signs. If further confirmation is needed, a blood test will show a rise in follicle stimulating hormone and luteinising hormone, and if the bones are badly affected, there will also be a rise in blood calcium and phosphates. A simple test which doctors can do is to examine some of the vaginal cells under a microscope; the cells with ample estrogen have dark well-marked nuclei within them. This is known as the Karyopicnotic Index (or K.I.), and is often done routinely when a cervical smear is performed, but its value is limited to the times when progesterone is absent, such as just after a period and after a long interval since the last period. If progesterone is present, the cells lose their nuclei.

If the diagnosis is in doubt it is worth giving the woman a month's trial of estrogen, and if on her return she reports an improvement in the symptoms the prescription can be repeated. Admittedly, there is frequently a beneficial placebo effect merely from giving the tablets, but if the improvement is still maintained two or three months later it strongly suggests that it is the hormone which is beneficial.

The effect of the menopause on sexual activity depends on one's experience during the menstruating years. If sex was important, then it is likely to be even more enjoyable once the fear of pregnancy is permanently eradicated. If there was never much sexual excitement, then many think of the menopause as a time when this activity may be slowed down or stopped. If estrogen deficiency is present and making the vagina sore and coital penetration painful, these symptoms can be easily relieved by giving estrogen, either as a cream to be used locally or as tablets.

Those who talk and write — in error — of the "male menopause," refer to it as a time when a man's sexual urge diminishes. This is nothing more than anti-chauvinism. It is also regrettable because it gives the impression that this is what is happening to women at menopause, which is quite wrong.

When Neuergarten was carrying out his study on attitudes toward menopause, he asked the loaded question, "What is the best thing about the menopause?" 44% replied "not having to bother about menstruation," 30% "not being worried about getting pregnant," and 14% "a better relationship with my husband and a greater enjoyment of sex life."

In 1969, the International Health Foundation studied the subject and interviewed 2,000 women aged between 45 and 55 years. 72% agreed that after menopause it was good to be free from menstruation. Figures for the various countries ranged from 66% in Italy to 79% in the United Kingdom.

EMPTY NEST SYNDROME

Unfortunately, the menopausal years are often traumatic for women in other ways. It has been calculated that in the space of the five years around her fiftieth birthday, the average woman will lose her mother through death, her daughter through marriage, and become a grandparent. There are also those homemakers whose children leave home for college or other employment, or who move because their husband changes his job or receives his final promotion. This has led psychologists to refer to the "Empty Nest Syndrome," believing that all the miseries of menopausal symptoms are but a reaction to the woman's empty life. While some women may be upset by these events, and the turmoil may cause emotional impulses to reach the menstrual clock, nevertheless, in the vast majority of cases the menopausal symptoms have a hormonal basis and respond well to estrogen therapy. Full details of treatment are to be found in Chapter 20.

19

Do It Yourself

There is a widespread hope that there may be some magic way of coping with monthly problems without having to disturb the busy doctor. Certainly, in mild cases it is important to try to tackle the problems yourself, with the full knowledge that if you do not succeed, further help — and the most effective help — is available from any doctor who understands hormone therapy.

First let us deal with the "old wives' tales," and remind you that there's no truth to the idea that you mustn't bathe, go swimming, or walk barefoot when you're menstruating or you will catch your death of cold. We now know that pneumonia commonly starts during the premenstruum, which is probably how the idea began. It won't matter if you do wash your hair when you're menstruating, although some women with very fine hair may find that a perm at this time of the month won't stay in for long. So if you're paying for an expensive perm, wait just a few days longer. Another false notion is that taking a cold shower will reduce the menstrual flow; this is wrong, for the menstrual flow is going to come normally, in its own good time.

The desire to "do-it-yourself" was expressed by a Community Nurse who wrote:

> "I always tended to be moody in my teens, but since my second pregnancy I have spells of hell, during which my doctor gives me tranquilizers. These help a bit, but as a state-registered nurse and health visitor, you can imagine my training screams out, 'Treat the cause, not the result.' Please tell me what I can do to help myself."

And from another nurse who pleaded:

> "There must be something more — I don't just want to take anti-depressants permanently when I feel so very well and am perfectly O.K. for half of the month."

RELAXATION AND BREATHING

For those with spasmodic dysmenorrhea, relaxation and correct breathing is valuable; unfortunately, the benefit is not so marked in those with premenstrual syndrome. It has been mentioned earlier that the type of pain suffered by those with severe spasmodic dysmenorrhea is similar to labor pains. Actually, the same nerves are involved in opening the door of the womb to let the baby out, as are needed at menstruation to open the door to let out the menstrual flow. Nowadays it is universally recognized that, in preparation for labor, women benefit by relaxation exercises and correct breathing. Gradually, it is being appreciated that these same relaxation exercises can also help to relieve the pain of dysmenorrhea. Some schools already teach older girls relaxation as part of physical education, and sufferers from dysmenorrhea have obtained much benefit from this. "Relaxation for Living" is an organization in Britain which exists purely to promote the teaching of relaxation, not only for that one day when the woman may be in labor, but to help both men and women to relax during their normal day-to-day living. The National Childbirth Trust runs classes throughout Britain for those who are pregnant, and are usually most helpful in supplying the name of a local teacher who will help either an individual or a group of girls with dysmenorrhea.

Drs. Margaret Chesney and Donald Tasto compared the effects of relaxation on college students in California. The students were initially separated into those with spasmodic dysmenorrhea and those with premenstrual syndrome; they were then divided into one of three treatment groups by drawing lots. One treatment group received relaxation treatment at five weekly sessions and was told to practice the exercises daily at home; another group attended a leaderless psychotherapy group where they compared each other's experiences of period pain for five weekly sessions; and the last group was left untreated. All students completed questionnaires dealing with the severity of their pain before treatment and for three cycles after treatment was completed. Those who had spasmodic dysmenorrhea and took relaxation classes reported a dramatic improvement in their condition, which was sustained afterward, but very few in the other groups benefited. So there does seem to be positive hope from simple treatment for those with spasmodic dysmenorrhea. However, if one is still being crippled with pain after thoroughly mastering the relaxation technique, there should be no hesitation in seeking help from the doctor, who can bring instant relief with a course of estrogen or prostaglandin inhibitors.

CHARTING YOUR SYMPTOMS

Sufferers from premenstrual syndrome will need different help. The first important thing is to keep a menstrual chart. You may devise your own, or use the types already described; it is the records which are important. If the chart shows the presence of symptoms during the paramenstruum, with freedom from symptoms during any other phase of the cycle, accept the diagnosis, and realize you are not alone; millions of other women are suffering likewise. Many letters received after a television program entitled *Pull Yourself Together, Woman* were from people who expressed this sense of relief:

> "I went to sleep happy that night knowing that I was not alone in my suffering."

> "Just to know I wasn't mad. I never dared talk about it; I thought I was the only one."

> "All my problems were so peculiar I didn't expect anyone else to understand."

What's more, you might even try charting a friend's problems, such as colds, accidents, or temper tantrums. Some people have complaints month after month and never link it up or make the connection with menstruation, they merely announce, "I've got another cold."

Having accepted the diagnosis yourself, talk about it. First, your husband should know and understand, so that he is able to help you. Wait until you feel well and then tell him how unhappy you feel about your periodic loss of control, and if it is relevant, about your fears that you might one day harm your baby or attempt an overdose. As mentioned earlier, sometimes when you feel most down during the premenstruum, you nevertheless have an increased sex urge. Discuss this with him, explain your difficulties, tell him that you know you're being awful but you can't help it, and you still love him and want him to love you. Having realized that there's nothing to be ashamed of, talk to the other people with whom you come into contact so that they may be able to understand you better. Discuss it with your friends so they can appreciate your difficulties and stand by you. Explain to your employer and to your in-laws, and don't forget it is just as important that men understand as well. Above all, see that your adolescent children understand and accept all that it entails. If you are at school, you should discuss it with your teacher, or if you are too shy you may want your mother to speak to the teacher instead.

During a Sunday family dinner, my adolescent daughter broke a plate when she was clearing away the first course. "Don't worry, it's the wrong day of the month," commented my son. Not many minutes later, my other daughter knocked over a glass and broke it. Trying to clear up the mess, I knocked a bowl of vegetables onto the floor. "I think we men will have to take care of the washing up today," remarked my other son calmly. It seemed a far better way of dealing with a biological disturbance than scolding the two girls for their apparent clumsiness.

Mark in your diary when you expect your next period. Don't assume 28 days just because others have a cycle of 28 days, but count the days of your last cycle and mark in the correct number of days for you personally. Consult your diary before arranging your next dinner party; avoid those awkward days if you have an interview, an examination or driving test. Arrange to have your perm or tint done during the postmenstrual week; it'll take better then. If you're a journalist, don't accept a deadline for any article which will clash with the worst time of the month. School teachers in high school can just as easily set homework two weeks ahead so that the girls can do it when in their postmenstrual peak. If you have to take examinations when you're feeling ill, make sure you tell the proctor, who should write a note on your paper telling the examiner.

If you're at work, tell your employer or your personnel manager. It helps if they understand. If flexitime is worked at your office, you'll be able to keep some hours or days in hand to use when necessary. If there is shift work, try to get on the midday shift so that you have time to get up without hurrying and dose yourself before starting the day's work. Sufferers from premenstrual syndrome should, if possible, avoid night shift work as nothing is more unsettling for the menstrual clock than mixing up night and day (remember the "sleep and waking" control center is also in the hypothalamus, near the menstrual clock). For the same reason, if you are going on a flight, be prepared to feel sleepy in the day and wakeful at night for a day or two after your journey.

EATING HABITS AND DIET

In Chapter 16 it was explained that, because the lower regulating mechanism for the control of blood sugar is raised premenstrually in sufferers of premenstrual syndrome, it is vital to ensure that long intervals without some starchy food are eliminated. The rule is to have small portions frequently, about every three hours. Instead of having two pieces of toast at breakfast, save one to enjoy with mid-morning coffee. Again, at lunch cut the sandwich (or whatever starchy food you usually have) into two, so that you have something to eat with your afternoon tea. And save something from your evening meal to enjoy before going to bed. It's really quite easy, and there's no need to eat more than your usual quantity.

Starchy food means anything made from flour, potatoes, rye, oats and rice, and therefore will include bread, cookies, crackers, potato chips and cereal, but be fully aware that it does not include fruit, chocolate and yogurt, which may be eaten with, but not instead of, starchy foods.

It is wise to always carry some emergency supplies of food in your handbag, ready for that long wait in line or the slow journey home. If your children are over five-years-old, tell them that the doctor says you must eat every three hours. It's amazing how cooperative children can be, always hoping that they too can enjoy a bite. Be sure your husband understands too, and ask him to give you a watch — or buy one yourself — which beeps when the three hours are up. It's essential to keep to the frequent snacks right through the cycle; it does no good just limiting it to the premenstruum.

It is useful to complete an attack form, shown in Figure 14, whenever you have a sudden attack of irritability, panic, or headache. It is surprising how often such problems start when there has been a food interval exceeding three hours. Incidentally, if you transgress and do inadvertently go too long without food, you may be surprised to find that it may take up to seven days to return to your normal level of fitness.

If you are good with your "three-hour rule" it is not necessary to limit your liquids drastically, but do not exceed two pints daily; similarly, it is safe to eat the normal amount of salt, but don't overdo it. See that your diet contains proteins and plenty of fruit and vegetables.

If you're going to indulge in alcohol, be warned that only half your usual amount will be required to make you merry. Intoxication can easily occur during the paramenstruum in sufferers from the premenstrual syndrome. It's as well to consider the other golden rules with regard to alcohol: don't mix grape and grain alcohol, or better still, don't mix your drinks; avoid drinking on an empty stomach; and don't drink and drive.

If constipation is a problem, or if you're unfortunate enough to have irritable bowel syndrome, then it is wise to add a tablespoon of bran to your breakfast every day. That is not quite the same as bran flakes or bran cereals. It is the natural bran that is important, the stuff that looks and tastes like sawdust. It cannot be enjoyed alone, but can be spread on your other cereals, added to fruit juice, yogurt or stewed fruit. Make it a daily habit, and after about two weeks you will appreciate its benefits with the regular, smooth opening of your bowels. In severe cases it may be necessary to have two tablespoons of bran daily, or have another helping of bran at night with cereals, soup, baked potatoes, stewed fruit or yogurt.

There is no evidence that premenstrual syndrome is caused by a poor diet or a deficiency of any known vitamin or mineral. Problems due to nutritional deficiencies, which can occur in men and women of all ages, will be present throughout the month, although, like all chronic diseases, the symptoms may be worse during the paramenstruum. Vitamins and minerals have no place in the treatment of premenstrual syndrome in those enjoying a healthy diet. The use of extra vitamins and minerals as self-medication is ill-advised, and can produce exacerbations or associated problems, as well as being useless and a waste of money.

It's a good idea to give yourself extra rest during the second half of the cycle and, if necessary, an afternoon nap too. Even if you don't go off to sleep, or into a state of semi-consciousness, it is resting in bed in the dark with the eyes shut that counts.

If a sufferer from premenstrual syndrome has taken all this advice and is still in trouble, I would have no hesitation in suggesting a visit to the doctor, appreciating that he has help at hand specifically for your problem. But remember to take your carefully prepared chart with you so that he, too, can confirm the diagnosis.

Finally, the menopausal woman, who is experiencing typical symptoms, would be well advised to avoid hot tea and coffee and spicy foods, in public anyway, as they do provoke hot flushes. Try to diet carefully, remembering that during this phase of life it is very easy for the fat ones to get fatter and the thin ones to get thinner. Ensure a good night's rest, which is not necessarily the same as a good night's sleep, by avoiding too many blankets which will only encourage the night sweats. If the nights are very disturbed, don't be ashamed of a short catnap after lunch. Your skin will also benefit from some cream to combat the natural dryness, and your greasy hair may need special shampoo.

20

What the Doctor Can Do

"How I resent those eight years of suffering now that I know how easy this is to cure."

"If only others knew that operations and being admitted to the hospital is not the answer to these beastly, savage changes of mood with the curse ... the real treatment is so simple."

The first step the doctor has to take when seeing a patient with menstrual problems is to ascertain the diagnosis, reassure himself that there is not some other accompanying disease, such as a non-related depressive illness, and convince himself that there is no evidence of malignancy.

"My doctor treats all of us with a D&C and that's it."

This comment may well be true, and merely shows how careful the doctor is being by first eliminating the possibility of cancer in the body of the womb, which would not show up on a cervical smear or pap smear. On the other hand, many gynecologists resort to the operation of dilatation and curettage at the drop of a hat, and such treatment can do nothing to cure any hormonal imbalance.

Having made sure of his diagnosis, the doctor now has to decide whether to use hormone therapy, and if so, which one. In this book we have been concerned essentially with the two menstrual hormones, estrogen and progesterone. Earlier chapters have shown how a deficiency of either of them will result in a completely different presentation of symptoms. To give progesterone to a woman suffering from spasmodic dysmenorrhea or menopausal symptoms will only make her worse, and the same happens when estrogens are given for premenstrual syndrome. This is why a definite diagnosis is essential before treatment can begin.

ESTROGEN THERAPY

The first estrogens to be used were non-steroidals, which had completely different formulas from the natural ones found in the body. These included stilbestrol, dioenestrol and hexoestradiol, which have been shown to have some cancer-producing potential and are rarely used today. The most important uses of estrogens are in the treatment of spasmodic dysmenorrhea, to help mature the womb in adolescence, to substitute for the failing of the ovarian estrogen at menopause, and in the contraceptive pill.

SPASMODIC DYSMENORRHEA

For many years, estrogens were the standard treatment for spasmodic dysmenorrhea, but our advancing knowledge that these women have high levels of prostaglandin F2 alpha has revolutionized treatment. Today, the drugs of choice are the prostaglandin inhibitors, which decrease the amount of prostaglandin in the tissues. These include ibuprofen (found in Advil, Motrin and Nuprin), mefanamic acid (Ponstel), indomethacin (Indocin), and naproxen (Naprosyn). Some are more specific against prostaglandin F2 alpha than others, which are more effective in reducing the prostaglandin released when bone cells are damaged. Mefanamic acid will both reduce the dysmenorrhea and also reduce the menstrual flow by about 25%. The tablets may be taken a day or two before menstruation is expected, and continued until the pain has eased. They can be obtained direct from the pharmacist without a doctor's prescription because their use is so safe.

If estrogen is being used, it is given in courses from day 5 for 21 days, and menstruation usually occurs within two days of stopping the tablets. The first course will result in painless menstruation because it has stopped ovulation for that month, but if one wants to remove spasmodic dysmenorrhea permanently, it is necessary to give many courses, perhaps for 6–12 months. In the 60s, when doing an investigation into period pains, it was surprising how many girls wrote that they had received one course of estrogens, which had only helped in that one month and made no difference thereafter. This is quite correct, but it is a shame that it was not pointed out to the girls when they started the treatment that more than one course would be necessary to remove the pain altogether.

The estrogen can either be given alone or mixed with progestogens, as in the estrogen-progestogen pill. The advantage of giving the pill is that one is sure menstruation will occur after 21 days and, of course, the pills are prepared in carefully dated packs of 21 so that they are not so easily forgotten, or if forgotten, the mistake is easily visible and two tablets can be taken at once when remembered. The advantage of giving estrogen alone is that varying amounts of estrogen can be given, thus allowing for individual variations. However, bleeding does not always occur at the end of the course. If estrogen is used alone, the girl must be fully aware that it is not a contraceptive.

> *Dierdre*, 19 years, had been given estrogen in Australia to relieve spasmodic dysmenorrhea. She went to Britain on a six-month holiday complete with sufficient tablets to last her stay. After about four months she realized she had missed her period, and began to develop morning sickness. Her pregnancy test proved positive.

As she was taking a pill every day for three weeks and stopping for one week, just like all her friends who were on the pill, she assumed hers was also a contraceptive.

Mothers are often upset by the thought that their daughters are being given the pill to ease period pains; they need to be reassured that this will not immediately lead their precious daughters up the path of rampant promiscuity. The girls also need to be reassured that, despite the terrible pains, their fertility is good, and the very fact of the pain shows that they are ovulating, so they should not have much trouble conceiving.

Occasionally, women asking for treatment of spasmodic dysmenorrhea are also anxious to begin a family. In these cases, it is worth giving a higher dose of estrogen from days 5 to 10 and days 18 to 28 of each cycle, avoiding estrogen at the time of ovulation so that conception can occur.

When estrogen is used for spasmodic dysmenorrhea before 25 years of age, side effects are rare because there is insufficient estrogen in the body and contraindications are hardly ever encountered.

ESTROGENS FOR MENOPAUSAL SYMPTOMS

When estrogens are given for menopausal symptoms, the effect is dramatic. A marked lessening in the number of daily flushes may be expected within a week, while if the flushes are still there in three weeks' time, it is a sign that a higher dose should be used. In Britain, prescriptions for estrogens have increased by 50% during the last four years, suggesting that its value is now being fully appreciated.

Women who are still menstruating can have estrogen from day 5 until the time of their expected menstruation. While for many women this may mean a three-week course, those with longer cycles would do better to have a longer course of estrogens. Otherwise they may have to go up to two weeks without treatment, and risk the return of all their symptoms.

It is suspected that the build-up of the lining of the womb in women who are not menstruating may be so marked that it could predispose them to cancer. No one really knows whether this is so, but there is a ready answer to this problem which is worth considering. The shedding of the lining can be induced by adding some progestogen, which is taken for a few days and then stopped. Bleeding is then likely to occur within a day or two of stopping. The progestogen can either be added to the estrogen tablet and taken daily for three weeks and then stopped for a week, during which bleeding will occur, or it may only be added for the last seven to ten days of the three weeks' course of estrogen. Some women may find that the added progestogens cause premenstrual syndrome, and these women benefit from the addition of oral progesterone instead of progestogens. This small amount of progesterone, which is absorbed orally, is sufficient to cause vaginal bleeding after a course of estrogen.

Those women who have had their womb removed and are suffering from menopausal symptoms will also benefit from estrogen therapy. They will not need to have the added progestogen, as there is no risk whatsoever of them developing cancer of the womb.

Estrogen can also be given through an implant, in which one or more small pellets of pure estrogen are inserted, under the influence of a local anesthetic, into the fat of the abdominal wall through a small incision in the skin. An implant means that the patient does not have the bother of trying to remember to take her daily tablets. It is particularly useful in women with menopausal symptoms who have had a hysterectomy in the past. An estrogen implant can also be performed for younger women during the course of their hysterectomy operation, in order to prevent too great a shock to their menstrual hormonal pathway. If there is any loss of libido, a pellet of testosterone implanted at the same time as the estrogen pellet will have a beneficial effect.

The estrogen replacement therapy should be continued until there are no symptoms when the estrogen is stopped. If the woman is having a three-week course of estrogen and has slight flushes during the week without treatment, she is not yet ready to stop. If she is free from symptoms then she can go for 10 days without starting the next course, and if all goes well, 14 days. If she can go three weeks without estrogen, it is a sign that her body has learned to make the estrogen necessary for healthy bone metabolism, and she can stop hormone replacement. Just how long it is necessary to continue treatment varies with the individual woman, and there are an unlucky few who may need to continue for 10 or more years.

Whether or not there is any risk in prolonged estrogen therapy is still a vexed question among the medical profession. Certainly, there does not appear to be a risk with short-term treatment. Follow-up studies of women who have had estrogen for 15 or more years are difficult and yield confusing results. In those days, many women had non-steroidal estrogens, which are known to carry a risk. However, we only hear of the cases where cancer develops, and we do not know whether this really represents all of the women in the sample who have been taking estrogen for a long time. Even women who have never had estrogen do develop cancer of the womb. Several long-term studies are in progress now, but it may be many years before a reliable answer is available.

Women on estrogen therapy should be seen at least every six months for a check on their blood pressure, weight and breasts, and for a general examination and cervical smear.

The side effects of estrogen are nausea, bloatedness, headaches and depression, but these will only occur with women in whom there is no estrogen deficiency, such as women with premenstrual syndrome.

At a recent meeting of a women's group, where a talk was being given on menopause, one member of the audience was very vocal and anxious to tell the audience that her doctor had refused to give her estrogen for her hot flushes. Later in the talk, mention was made of the indications for avoiding estrogens. These include a past history of coronary thrombosis; angina; pulmonary embolism; deep vein thrombosis; cancer of the breast, womb or ovary; diabetes; liver disease; and high blood pressure. The same woman then rose and apologized, as she was under treatment for high blood pressure.

Some doctors feel that by eliminating the menstrual cycle they can also eliminate premenstrual syndrome; unfortunately, it is not as easy as that, for as we have noted, cyclical symptoms still occur after a hysterectomy and oophorectomy. Some advocate an estrogen implant to abolish menstruation, and then the addition of progestogens at the beginning of each month to ensure that there is regular shedding of the lining of the womb. The menstrual cycle of women who undergo such treatment is disturbed for up to one year and symptoms occur throughout the cycle. Their symptom-free postmenstruum is abolished.

TREATMENT FOR
PREMENSTRUAL SYNDROME

A woman journalist conducted a small private survey to find

out what other doctors were doing about menstrual problems. She noted the following as pretty standard answers.

"It (progesterone) doesn't work, and anyway, everybody's on the pill."

"It can only be given by injections."

"There is no proof it works."

"Placebo effects."

"Women are supposed to get some kind of masochistic pleasure from their pains."

There is nothing very surprising about these comments, for they are typical of the attitudes which are delaying, for many premenstrual syndrome sufferers, the relief to which they are entitled. The first one is typical of the confusion in many doctors' minds between progesterone and progestogens. Progestogens do not work on premenstrual syndrome, progesterone does. The confusion is reinforced by the statement that follows, "everybody's on the pill." The next comment is from those who may know the difference but are unaware of the progress that has been made with suppositories and pessaries. The third remark is symptomatic of our scientific age, which cannot accept the evidence of its own eyes without the support of strictly controlled clinical trials. "The proof of the pudding lies in the eating," or so it is said. The women whose quotes appeared at the beginning of this chapter needed no further proof of its value in treating premenstrual syndrome other than their own satisfactory experience. The other remarks need no comment; indeed, they are all rather like doctors' old wives' tales. In fairness to the doctors, it must be remembered that not many who are practicing today were taught anything about these hormones when they were at medical school. But there are increasing numbers of doctors today who do know how and when to use estrogen and progesterone to remove the monthly sufferings of women.

PROGESTERONE

The first person to use the word "progesterone" was Willard Allen, who, with George Corner, first isolated the active constituent of the corpus luteum in the ovary. He proposed the name in December 1934, and eight months later the principal scientists involved in work on this new female sex hormone accepted the name. In 1943, Russell Marker emerged from the jungles of Central America and showed biochemists how to manufacture this pregnancy hormone — progesterone — from the roots of yams. However, once the biochemists had learned the knack of manufacturing progesterone from yams, its own importance was overshadowed by the many other steroids that could be obtained from it just by a subtle alteration of its chemical formula. In their laboratories, the biochemists converted progesterone into the life-saving hormone, cortisone, and it was also converted into progestogens, which are the basis of oral contraceptives and are used by countless women the world over. Progesterone is also converted into estrogens for use in hormone replacement therapy, and into testosterone for the restoration of male potency.

PROGESTERONE THERAPY

For many doctors, progesterone is a forgotten hormone as far as treatment is concerned. Many doctors who use estrogen and know its possibilities and limitations are shy of using progesterone. One problem is that progesterone taken orally is not effective in the treatment of premenstrual syndrome, so it has to be given in other ways. These include suppositories that can be inserted into the rectum or vagina, injections or implants. In India, work on monkeys suggested that progesterone could be absorbed into the blood stream when given nasally, so aerosols and nasal sprays were tried but with little success. Later, it was shown that progesterone cream applied to the noses of female rats was well absorbed. An American pharmaceutical company, Nastech, reported in 1985 that tests have been carried out on women in North Carolina and in

Yorkshire, England, in which progesterone nasal cream has been used with satisfactory results. There are hopes that this method of administration may revolutionize future progesterone therapy.

When a woman with premenstrual syndrome who has been treated with progesterone returns to the doctor, it is often difficult to recognize her as the same person who first came for advice and treatment. The woman who so often took an overdose of barbiturates during the late premenstruum, when life was on top of her, will return delighted and tell you of the interesting evening classes she is now attending. The alcoholic, who used to get herself into trouble each month, will discuss the dream holiday she is planning. The husband comes in to tell you about his wife "who is now the woman I married." There is the mother who is so delighted because "even the children are behaving nowadays," and the student who has happily passed her final examinations, the epileptic mother whose children are once more returned home to her care, and the asthmatic who drove to London Bridge to ceremoniously throw overboard her now redundant aerosol inhalers. For women who have suffered some of the serious consequences of premenstrual syndrome that we have discussed in earlier chapters, it is really no hardship to have to administer their progesterone by pessary, suppository or injection, instead of the more conventional way through the mouth.

PROGESTERONE SUPPOSITORIES

Progesterone suppositories are small pellets of inert wax containing progesterone which are inserted into the vagina or rectum. The wax melts at body temperature, releasing the progesterone, which is absorbed through the lining of the vagina or rectum and conveyed in the blood to where it is needed. The wax is expelled from the body, either moistening the vagina or mixed with the feces. Women who have vaginal infections are invariably treated with suppositories, and there are rarely any complaints. Suppositories are easy enough to insert into the anus, and were used by the ancient Egyptians, Greeks and Romans for the administration of drugs to the rectum, where they are easily absorbed into the bloodstream. They have, however, never been a popular method of treatment in Anglo-Saxon countries and America.

During a recent vacation in Spain, we were enjoying a pleasant evening with our Spanish hosts when their four-year-old daughter emerged into the lounge complaining she could not go to sleep because of an earache. The mother searched in her handbag and gave the little one a suppository, probably a pain-reliever, which she took away and apparently used herself quite satisfactorily. Women who have learned to appreciate the value of progesterone no longer object to using suppositories.

Many years of research preceded the introduction of commercially produced progesterone suppositories. The base in which the progesterone was dissolved had to be carefully selected, as the original ones tended to cause irritation and diarrhea. Regulation of the temperature appeared important while preparing the suppositories to prevent the formation of crystals, which produced painful pricking sensations when inserted. If the suppository melted at too high a temperature, those women with low body temperatures complained of grittiness.

In practice, rectal or vaginal suppositories are interchangeable; it is usually left to the individual to select the one she prefers, and she may use both on alternate occasions. Patients are given permission to use an extra suppository when an unexpected need arises, such as when a sudden surge of irritability is building up or an impending migraine threatens. Up to six 400mg suppositories can be used in a day; after all, during pregnancy the blood level of progesterone is so high that it would take 30 suppositories daily to reach the same level. If two suppositories are used simultaneously in the same orifice, the melted wax prevents further absorption of progesterone, so it is impossible for an individual to overdose with suppositories. It is important to advise women not to insert a tampon at the same time as the suppository, otherwise the tampon absorbs the progesterone and the woman receives no benefit.

The time of giving progesterone will be determined by observing each individual patient's chart. In the normal case, it is given as suppositories from midcycle until the onset of menstruation. However, if symptoms continue until the second or third day of menstruation, then the progesterone should be continued until the fourth day. If symptoms start at ovulation, the progesterone should be started a couple of days beforehand. In short, the program should be individually tailored for each patient. The progesterone needs to be started at midcycle, or at least four days before the symptoms are expected, and continued until menstruation has started. It is quite useless to give suppositories on alternate days from day 19 to 25, which is how it was given in the double-blind controlled test reported by S. L. Smith (1975), which is often quoted to claim that progesterone is ineffective because it was unsuccessful in that particular trial. The progesterone could never have demonstrated its effectiveness for it was used too late, without regard for individual variation in the length of cycle, for too short a time, and with too long an interval between each administration of progesterone.

There is a marked variation in the absorption of progesterone by individuals — some absorb quickly and others more slowly, some show immediate increases in the blood progesterone level and in others, the rise or fall is slower. Furthermore, there is a small proportion of women, between 5% and 10%, who do not absorb progesterone effectively from the rectum or vagina, and who will need progesterone by injection. The absorption of suppositories is usually quick, and within 20 minutes there may be a rise in the level of progesterone in the blood, but the progesterone level may drop quite quickly too, and the effect is always over within 24 hours. In some women the effect only lasts four hours. This means that some women may need to take 2–6 suppositories daily.

PROGESTERONE INJECTIONS

Progesterone injections last longer than suppositories. In some women, they only need to be repeated on alternate days, while others need them daily. The absorption is more reliable, and so they are used in desperate situations, such as when a marriage is at a breaking point, or children are in danger of being taken away. Another advantage is that if they are given daily by a nurse, she can silently supervise those who need watching in the premenstruum — for instance, where there is a risk of suicide, child abuse or excessive drinking. Injections are more convenient for patients in hospitals and are also used where suppositories have failed.

At first the injections are given by a nurse, but with suitable instruction, most patients soon learn the art of giving their own. Failing this, the husband may be ready to learn the technique. In the buttocks, between the muscles and fibers, there are clumps of fat cells which form a cushion for us to sit on. The progesterone injection should be inserted into the buttock muscles, where it is absorbed by the fat cells and then gradually released into the blood. The injections should not be given into the thigh or arm, where there are no fat cells between the muscle fibers. The injection can be given anywhere in the buttocks where there is a one-inch pinch of flesh, which means it cannot be given in the upper inner quadrant where the skin is closely attached to the end of the spine.

PROGESTERONE IMPLANT

Progesterone can also be given by implants to those who have already had complete relief of symptoms with either suppositories or injections. This relieves the need for daily medication and lasts for an average of 3–4 months, and occasionally for as long as 18 months. It is particularly useful for women who have had their womb removed, as they will not be troubled by the erratic menstruation which sometimes follows. It is also used for those who are forgetful in giving themselves progesterone, such as irresponsible alcoholics or drug users. One patient living in Italy calculated that the cost of an annual implant, plus the air fare from Rome, was cheaper than the cost of daily suppositories.

However, a progesterone implant is not as convenient as an estrogen implant. More progesterone pellets are used, and they sometimes have a tendency to be extruded, or pushed out. Incidents of extrusion are likely to occur at times of greatest progesterone need, such as during the pre-menstruum. The site of the implant becomes inflamed, but this can be eased by giving progesterone injections for five consecutive days, thus temporarily giving the body an alterna-tive supply of progesterone.

A progesterone implant should not be given to those hoping to conceive within 12 months; those unduly con-cerned when their normal menstruation is replaced by an irregular scanty loss or possibly missed menstruation for up to six months; those who must avoid premenstrual symptoms at all costs, such as the epileptic woman who may not realize that her implanted supply of progesterone is running low and has an epileptic attack at a most unfortunate or potentially dangerous time; and those whose normal daily requirement of progesterone is very high.

If progesterone is given daily by pessaries, suppositories or injections and then stopped for some reason, menstruation will occur. This is similar to what happens when the level of progesterone drops and menstruation occurs in a normal cycle.

It is impossible to give an overdose of progesterone to a woman who has borne children, because during pregnancy women are exposed to a thirtyfold increase in their blood progesterone level for nine full months, instead of just a mere two weeks, and the body has learned to deal with that. On the other hand, in childless and immature women an excess of progesterone may occasionally cause euphoria, rest-less energy, insomnia and dysmenorrhea or uterine cramps similar to those suffered in spasmodic dysmenorrhea.

There are no contraindications for the use of proges-terone. Also, there are no risks of progesterone causing can-cer. In fact, progesterone is used in the treatment of some cancers, especially those produced in the vaginas of teenage girls who were exposed to stilbestrol (DES) during their fetal life, and advanced or recurrent cancer of the womb. If there is any possibility of candida (yeast infections) being present, this should be cleared up before pessaries are used, as proges-terone may encourage candida to grow.

Progesterone suppositories in doses of 200mg and 400mg are commercially available in Britain under the trade name of

"Cyclogest," distributed and marketed by Hoechst U.K. Ltd. For many years, the Food and Drug Administration in the United States has permitted the commercial production of progesterone injections and also of 50mg progesterone suppositories for infertility patients with luteal phase deficiency of progesterone. Tests are now proceeding for the use of higher doses of progesterone. In Britain, progesterone suppositories of 200mg and 400mg have been available for 20 years and, in my personal experience, several thousand women have been using them for many years. Meanwhile, in the United States it is quite legal for any pharmacist to make up progesterone suppositories of any strength on a doctor's prescription for a specific patient.

PROGESTOGENS

Because progesterone cannot be given by mouth, biochemists sought for a synthetic preparation which could be absorbed orally. They tried making small alterations to the chemical formula, hoping to find one with slightly different properties; after all, the formulae of progesterone, estrogen, testosterone and cortisone are all very similar, although they have quite different properties. The biochemists succeeded in finding the progestogens, which are the basis of all contraceptive pills, and gave rise to a multimillion dollar industry. When the progestogens were first discovered, it was believed that they were true progesterone substitutes. But, in effect, they had some properties of estrogen, some of progesterone, and some of testosterone. If progestogens have been given during pregnancy, and the child is a girl, she is likely to show masculinizing effects in her genitals and be a tom-boy, with marked aggression. This is quite different from the effect of natural progesterone, which is produced in such large quantities during pregnancy. Indeed, surveys have suggested that if progesterone is given to mothers before the sixteenth week of pregnancy for eight weeks or longer, the child of that pregnancy has a tendency toward an enhanced intelligence, with a good academic record, higher grades, and a better chance of reaching university level than control children whose mothers

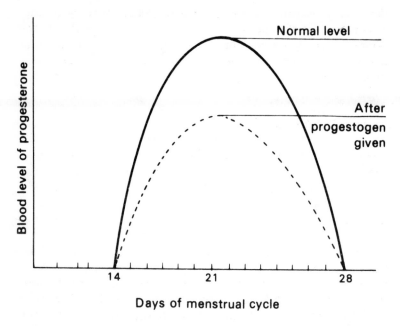

Figure 34   Effect of progestogen on the blood level of progesterone

were not given progesterone.

There are many differences between progesterone and the various progestogens, but unfortunately there are still some doctors who do not realize this. Progesterone lowers the blood pressure while progestogens raise it, and whereas progesterone raises SHBG, progestogens lower it. Progestogens are not used by progesterone receptors. Progesterone can relieve water and sodium retention whereas some progestogens used in the pill, such as nor-ethisterone, cause a retention of water and sodium. Progesterone is converted by the adrenals into all the various corticosteroids, which is not possible with progestogens. The function of progesterone is also to maintain a pregnancy, but the progestogens cannot be used for this purpose. Some progestogens have an estrogenic effect as well, which is useful in the contraceptive field.

Some doctors believe that by eliminating ovulation and menstruation with the use of strong progestogens, such as danazol, it is possible to eliminate premenstrual syndrome. Unfortunately, this does not occur — it merely prolongs the premenstrual symptoms throughout the cycle. On the other hand, danazol is often the drug of choice in the treatment of endometriosis.

CONTRACEPTION

For those who have or have had spasmodic dysmenorrhea, the estrogen-progestogen pill is usually the best method of contraception. These women have a low estrogen level and benefit when given some extra estrogen. In fact, many of them were unhappy when the high estrogen pills were removed from the market, because they felt so much better on a high dose. On the other hand, premenstrual syndrome sufferers tend to have difficulty with the pill, which causes an increase in headaches, weight-gain, depression and nausea; they are also candidates for the more serious blood clotting problems. Furthermore, the progestogens tend to lower the normal progesterone level, making their premenstrual syndrome worse.

Unfortunately, intra-uterine contraceptive devices (IUDs) have a tendency, in some women, to make menstruation heavier or longer, and are therefore best avoided by those who already have heavy periods.

Women who are receiving progesterone treatment for premenstrual syndrome can take a progestogen-only pill from day 1 until day 11 and then start the normal progesterone dose until menstruation. Or they can start with a small amount of progesterone, say a 50mg progesterone suppository, from day 8, and take that until they start their normal course of progesterone and continue it up to the start of menstruation. In this way, they are contraceptively safe. Progesterone is nature's own contraceptive; it is present after ovulation and converts the thin vaginal mucus into a thick, sticky type which prevents sperm from entering the womb.

Sterilization is not the ultimate and universal answer to the problem of contraception, for women with premenstrual syndrome may find the operation increases their symptoms (see page 28). Recently, B.W. McGuiness, a family doctor in Cheshire, England, in a controlled series of tests, found that women who have bilateral tubal ligation suffered significantly more menstrual cycle disturbances post-operatively.

CONCEPTION

Those women on progesterone treatment who are anxious to conceive are advised to start their progesterone 48 hours after their temperature chart shows ovulation has occurred. If they do not know when ovulation occurs they should start on day 16 for cycles of up to 28 days, and on day 18 for longer cycles. They should be advised to continue the progesterone until the pregnancy is confirmed, and then only to stop if they are free from pregnancy symptoms.

TESTOSTERONE

Testosterone, the male hormone, has occasionally been used for the treatment of premenstrual syndrome, especially in those who have sore breasts premenstrually. It is effective, especially in giving energy, lightening or stopping menstruation, and easing the engorged breasts. However, it can have masculinizing effects such as hoarseness, a deepening of the voice and the growing of hair on the beard area of the face. Testosterone is also valuable in rapidly stopping menopausal flushes and depression when it is given in a combined tablet with estrogen. This may be useful during the initial treatment for a month or two in a severely ill patient at the menopause. Testosterone also improves the sex urge and activity, and may be used in implants together with estrogen.

BROMOCRIPTINE

Bromocriptine is a drug which is capable of lowering a raised prolactin level. As explained in Chapter 15, sometimes a raised prolactin level interferes with the progesterone feedback pathway from the womb to the hypothalamus. There are reports from Holland that patients with infertility and premenstrual syndrome have been successfully treated with bromocriptine. However, strictly controlled tests on patients in England carried out by Ghose and Coppen, using a different dosage, have not confirmed these findings. Patients who appear to benefit from bromocriptine are those with marked water retention, painful and engorged breasts, those who have lost their sex interest, those who have recently had postnatal depression, and women with raised prolactin levels.

PYRIDOXINE

Pyridoxine, or vitamin B 6, has been recommended for women who become depressed when using estrogen-progestogen contraception, and also for menopausal women receiving estrogen replacement therapy. Unfortunately, worldwide clinical tests have failed to show the value of pyridoxine in women with well-diagnosed premenstrual syndrome. The recommended daily requirement of B 6 is only 2–4 mg, yet doses of 10 or even 100 times that amount are often prescribed. Increasingly, since 1983, symptoms of pyridoxine overdose have been observed. In some sensitive women, symptoms of overdose may occur within a few months of taking pyridoxine, but it is more usual for it to occur when excessive amounts have been taken for three or more years. Nor does it matter whether pyridoxine is taken alone, with other B vitamins, with other vitamins, or with magnesium; the incidence of symptoms of overdose is the same. The early symptoms of overdose are depression, headache, tiredness, bloatedness and irritability. One or more of these symptoms may have been present before pyridoxine was started and becomes more severe. At a later stage, there is a numbness with pins and needles in the arms, legs and face, tingling, burning and creeping sensations in the skin, shooting pains and muscle weakness. As the symptoms progress, the muscle weakness makes typing difficult, fine needlework is no longer possible, and walking becomes difficult, until finally, a walking cane and then wheelchair is needed. Fortunately, when

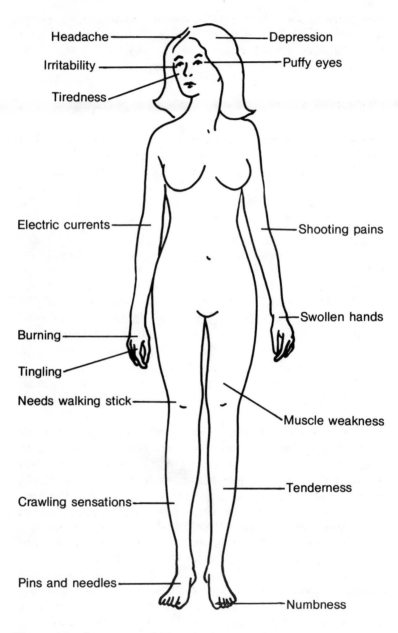

Figure 35   Symptoms of Vitamin B 6 overdose

pyridoxine is abruptly stopped, there are no withdrawal symptoms, no further progression, and a gradual recovery from the temporary disabilities.

CLONIDINE

Clonidine, marketed under the name of Dixarit, is a drug used for lowering blood pressure, and in very small doses it may be used to relieve menopausal flushes in those who, for some reason, are unable to tolerate estrogens. However, it only acts on the flushes and is of no value in relieving the other estrogen-deficiency symptoms at the menopause, such as vagina and skin thinning, joint pains and psychological symptoms. One beautiful menopausal lady, who always had a perfectly coiffured head of white hair, refused to have a further course of estrogens, which, although they cured her menopausal flushes and depression, caused some of her white hairs to become grey again. She opted for Clonidine, at least for a few months, until the psychological symptoms bore down on her.

DIURETICS

It is best to avoid diuretics, as any help they give to those with water retention is only temporary, and it is so easy to repeat them indefinitely, always taking more and more until the balance of sodium and potassium is disturbed. Diuretics do not help the premenstrual tension, depression or irritability, only the symptoms due to water retention, such as bloatedness, gain in weight and swollen ankles. Once addicted to diuretics, it is difficult to stop taking them. It must be done gradually, first reducing from four to three, then three to two at monthly intervals, always reducing in the postmenstruum. When the dose is down to one daily, the reduction should continue, taking the diuretic on alternate days, then every third day and every fourth day, until it is finally stopped.

POTASSIUM

A lowering of the blood potassium level may be suspected in those who have been taking diuretics for a long time, those who have food cravings and prolonged dieting, and those who complain of exhaustion and muscle weakness throughout the cycle. These women should have a blood potassium estimation and, if necessary, be given potassium tablets regularly.

21

A Fairer Future

This book is written with the aim of spreading the news to mankind that the once-a-month miseries of countless women can be, and are being, successfully treated and relieved. At the same time, it is hoped that it will help men to understand and appreciate the menstrual problems of women, and become partners in helping them through their difficult days. That you are reading this brings hope that the aim will be achieved.

Menstrual miseries are widespread and incapacitating at times; their effects can involve all classes, all ages, and both sexes. Nevertheless, it is possible to abolish dysmenorrhea, premenstrual syndrome and menopausal problems by giving hormone treatment. But although treatment is possible, it is not yet universal. Menopausal clinics are now well-established and countrywide gynecological help is available for the relief of symptoms related to the change of life. The recognition of premenstrual syndrome is not yet as widespread, although since the first edition of this book there have been some encouraging developments. For a list of clinics, support and information groups in the U.S.A. see p. 214.

In 1983, Mrs. Lindsay Burton Leckie and Mrs. Pat Cannon, both of whom suffered from premenstrual syndrome and both of whom had benefitted from progesterone therapy, founded the National PMS Society, a non-profit, all-volunteer, educational and support network consisting of 91 affiliated groups throughout the United States. Their goals are to educate the medical and lay community in the identification and treatment of premenstrual syndrome, to promote among the general public an awareness of the existence of premenstrual

193

syndrome, and to assist women by offering emotional support and up-dated information. This information is available through the Society's own literature and newsletters as well as other literature on premenstrual syndrome. Other activities include walk-in counseling, telephone hotlines, public meetings, workshops and seminars, and fund-raising for premenstrual syndrome research.

Premenstrual syndrome really should be a specialty of general practice, and should be mastered by every general practitioner. The day will surely come when every general practitioner and consultant is able to diagnose, treat and manage all cases of premenstrual syndrome which come within his or her orbit. The long-term follow-up of a chronic disease such as premenstrual syndrome is best done by a general practitioner, who is the physician of continuing care, rather than in hospitals, with their ever-changing junior staff and their need to discharge patients as soon as possible to make way for new ones. At present, however, this goal is a long way off.

The gynecologist tends to be satisfied with a faultless physical examination and the reassurance of a "D& C," and is then content to refer the patient back to the family doctor. The endocrinologists have more serious diseases to occupy their time and rarely wish to be troubled by disturbances of menstrual hormones, especially at a time when there are not enough useful hormonal estimations to clinch the diagnosis and determine the dosage of hormones needed. Psychiatrists do occasionally recognize the syndrome and prescribe antidepressants or tranquilizers, but they next see the patient in the symptom-free postmenstruum and discharge her from their care. Neurologists fully investigate all cases of epilepsy and migraine to satisfy themselves that no lesion is present, and then discharge the patient. The chest physician treats the asthma, the rhinologist the allergic rhinitis, the orthopedic surgeon and rheumatologist the backache and painful joints, the dermatologist the herpes and neurodermatitis, but even if all the menstrually-related symptoms are appreciated by these consultants, the overall diagnosis is still too easily ignored.

If Premenstrual Syndrome Clinics are to be established, the general practitioner will need to be in the forefront, assisted by a psychiatrist and gynecologist, for it is only the general practitioner who encompasses the whole vista of symptoms and knows the effect on the family. Before he is ready to accept this role the general practitioner needs specialized courses in diagnosing and treating these menstrual problems, and medical students require a greater familiarity with the subject during their undergraduate training. The general practitioner needs to know the art of adjusting menstruation for vital events, knowing the methods and their hazards, the utilization of the peak postmenstrual days, and how to recognize those women with dysmenorrhea and premenstrual syndrome who urgently need treatment.

In Great Britain, in 1985, the National Commission for Women called the attention of the Cabinet to the need for greater undergraduate and postgraduate education on premenstrual syndrome, and the need for training teachers, social workers, police and lawyers about this subject.

The need for greater public education and awareness is obvious, and here is an opportunity to be grasped by the media and offered to a public always hungry for human interest stories and news of medical possibilities. But we must remember that doctors do not like to be told by the popular press what treatment they should give their patients. Education on these subjects should extend to schools, where both sexes should be made aware of the problems and the solutions which are at hand.

It is estimated that the cost of menstrual problems to American industry is equal to 8% of the total wages paid. Would it not be better for industry to invest a fraction of that sum in menstrual clinics and training schemes for doctors, in order to speed the time when such wastage will be eliminated?

School and university examinations can be made fairer by adjusting the timetable so that exams are set a week apart, by having compulsory questions in all tests rather than one compulsory exam, by setting alternative dates where possible, and by offering a choice of dates for practical and oral examinations. Teachers can set the pupils' work two or more weeks in advance.

A greater appreciation of the relationship of premenstrual syndrome to social and domestic violence would enable premenstrual baby battering to be correctly diagnosed, under-

stood and treated, thereby eliminating the problem and re-
moving the social stigmas of separation, children being taken
into care, and criminal proceedings.

The ideal would seem to be to abolish menstruation
altogether at those times when conception is not required.
This can be done by the prolonged administration of progestogens, but it is not yet ideal. Initially there tends to be the
occasional breakthrough bleeding, and then after a year or
two, there is a subtle change in the personality of the woman:
she becomes harder and more efficient, with loss of sex
interest. Is the price worth it? Already there is the technique
of menstrual aspiration, which women can learn to perform
themselves, in which they suck the menstrual flow from the
womb through a thin flexible plastic tube and complete menstruation in one minute or less. Unfortunately, menstrual
hormones may be upset by this event and their smooth ebb
and flow drastically altered. The layman, or rather laywoman,
too eagerly hopes that the mere removal of the womb will
accomplish the feat, but as has already been discussed, the
removal of the womb too often upsets the hormonal pathway, and the end result may be worse than the condition
before the operation.

In the last century, essayist John Ruskin reminded his
fellow countrymen that "the true wealth of the Nation was
running to waste" because most children had no sort of
education. The same could be said today about the lack of
education and understanding about premenstrual syndrome.
Discussion of menstruation and its attendant problems should
be as open and unrestricted as the discussion of sex, and the
knowledge and understanding of menstruation should be available to all.

Having read as far as this, there will probably be two nagging questions in your mind. "If progesterone and estrogen
are so successful in their respective treatments, why aren't
more doctors using them?" and, "Why do some doctors prefer to use a drug which is less successful and only brings partial relief to a portion of patients with mild symptoms, rather
than one which brings complete relief to most patients with
mild and severe symptoms?"

There is no simple answer to these perfectly reasonable

questions. Some answers are contained in earlier chapters, but there are a number of other reasons which can be grouped under three broad headings:

1) Doctors have an essentially conservative approach.

2) Commercial aspects.

3) Lack of consultancy and treatment facilities.

Very few of the doctors in practice today have had any training in diagnosing or treating what we now know as the world's most common disease, premenstrual syndrome. Doctors are themselves wholly responsible for the diagnosis and treatment of their patients, and they alone have the right to protect their patients as well as themselves; therefore, they have a natural reticence about using treatments which they are not yet fully persuaded are safe and effective. However, this does place on them the responsibility for increasing their knowledge of the subject, for the average general practitioner will have in his practice some 50 women with premenstrual syndrome needing treatment.

In today's world one cannot overlook commercial pressures. Progesterone has no protective patent, and therefore no American drug manufacturer will benefit financially from marketing it. The cost of clinical trials and of gathering the necessary evidence to convince the F.D.A. of the efficacy of progesterone in the treatment of premenstrual syndrome is prohibitive, and if any manufacturer were to succeed in getting a license, there is no guarantee of a profit, for any other manufacturer would be free to produce a similar product. On the other hand, vitamins and minerals are a good source of profit and can be advertised to the general public and sold over the counter without a medical prescription. However, they are no more beneficial to women with premenstrual syndrome than to healthy men, women and children.

The general practitioner who has a patient with a condition he does not understand, will forward that patient to a consultant who specializes in that particular problem. But to whom will we send the case of premenstrual asthma or premenstrual sinusitis, which has been confirmed by a menstrual chart? Not to a gynecologist or endocrinologist or psychiatrist.

These are but partial answers to our two questions, but it must be appreciated that the number of doctors who can diagnose and treat these menstrual problems increases all the time. If more clinics could be established and training courses instituted, the number of undiagnosed and untreated sufferers would steadily decrease.

A quotation from Henry David Thoreau runs:

> "If you have built
> Castles in the air,
> Your work need
> Not be lost;
> There is where they
> Should be.
> Now put foundations under them."

Let us get down to work.

Other Publications
by the Author

The Premenstrual Syndrome (1953), Joint authorship R. Greene. Brit. Med. J., 1, 1007.

The Similarity of Symptomatology of Premenstrual Syndrome and Toxaemia of Pregnancy and their Response to Progesterone (1954) (Charles Oliver Hawthorne BMA Prize Essay), Brit. Med. J., 1, 1071.

Comparative Trials of New Oral Progestogenic Compounds in Treatment of Premenstrual Syndrome (1959), ibid., 2, 1307–1309.

The Premenstrual Syndrome (1955), Proceedings of the Royal Society of Medicine, 48, 5, 337.

The Aftermath of Hysterectomy and Oophorectomy (1957), Proc. Roy. Soc. Med., 50, 6, 415–418.

Menstruation and Acute Psychiatric Illnesses (1959), Brit. Med. J., 1, 148.

Effect of Menstruation on Schoolgirls' Weekly Work (1960), ibid., 1, 326–328.

Menstruation and Accidents (1960), ibid., 2, 1425.

Schoolgirls' Behaviour and Menstruation (1960), ibid., 2, 1647–1649.

Menstruation and Crime (1961), ibid., 2, 1752.

The Influence of Menstruation on Health and Disease (1964), Proc. Roy. Soc. Med., 57, 4, 262.

THE PREMENSTRUAL SYNDROME (1964), London: William Heinemann Medical Books.

The Influence of Mother's Menstruation on her Child (1966) (Charles Oliver Hawthorne BMA Prize Essay), Proc. Roy. Soc. Med., 59, 10, 1014–1016.

The Influence of Menstruation on Glaucoma (1967) (Charles Oliver Hawthorne BMA Prize Essay), Brit. J. Ophthal., 51, 10, 692.

Ante-Natal Progesterone and Intelligence (1968), Brit. J. Psych., 516, 114, 1377.

Menstruation and Examinations (1968), Lancet, 11, 1386.

THE MENSTRUAL CYCLE (1969), London: Penguin Books.

Children's Hospital Admissions and Mother's Menstruation (1970), Brit. Med. J., 2, 27–8.

Migraine in General Practice (1973) (Migraine Trust Prize Essay), J. Roy. Coll. Gen. Pract., 23, 97.

Effect of Progesterone on Brain Function (1975), X Acta Endocrin. Congr., Amsterdam.

Sexual and Menstrual Problems in the Blind (1976), Conference of Sexual Problems of the Disabled, Royal College of Obstetricians and Gynaecologists, London.

Migraine and Oral Contraceptives (1976), Headache, 15, 4, 247.

Menstruation and Sport (1976), Chapter in SPORTS MEDICINE, 2nd Edition, Ed. J. P. R. Williams & P. N. Sperrin, Edward Arnold, London.

Prenatal Progesterone and Educational Attainments (1976) (Charles Oliver Hawthorne BMA Prize Essay), Brit. J. Psych., November, 129, 438.

PREMENSTRUAL SYNDROME AND PROGESTERONE THERAPY (1977, 2nd Ed. 1984), London: William Heinemann Medical Books Ltd.; Chicago: Year Book Medical Publishers Inc.

Menarcheal Age in the Disabled (1978), Joint authorship with Maureen E. Dalton. Brit. Med. J., 2, 475.

Cyclical Criminal Acts in Premenstrual Syndrome (1980), Lancet, 1070–1071.

DEPRESSION AFTER CHILDBIRTH (1980, 2nd Ed. 1984), London: Oxford University Press.

The Legal Implications of Premenstrual Syndrome (1982), World Medicine, 17th April 1982.

Overview of Premenstrual Tension (1982), Chapter 11 in MENSTRUATION AND BEHAVIOUR, Ed. R. Friedman, Marcel Dekker, New York.

What is this PMS? (1982), J. Roy. Col. Gen. Pract., 717–719.

Premenstrual Syndrome: A New Criminal Defense? (1982), Joint authorship with Laurence Taylor. Calif. West. Law Rev., 19, 2, 269–287.

Premenstrual Syndrome and its Treatment (1983), International Medicine.

Progesterone Prophylaxis used successfully in Postnatal Depression (1985), Practitioner, 229, 507.

Menstrual Stress (1985), Stress Medicine Vol. 1, 127–133.

Legal Implications of PMS (1986), Hamline Law Review, 9, 1, 143–154.

Vitamins: a new Prospective (1986), Mims Magazine, 15th March, 1986.

Should Premenstrual Syndrome be a Legal Defence? (1986), Chapter in PREMENSTRUAL SYNDROME: ETHICAL IMPLICATIONS IN A BIO-BEHAVIOURAL PROSPECTIVE, Ed. B. F. Carter & B. E. Ginsburg, (pub-date 1986).

Glossary

Adrenal glands — two glands situated above the kidney and responsible for producing numerous hormones.

Adrenalin — one of the many hormones produced by the adrenal glands.

Analgesics — pain relievers.

Anovular — without ovulation.

Ante-natal — before childbirth.

Cervical smear — test for the diagnosis of cancer of the neck of the womb.

Cervix — neck of the womb.

Climacteric — change of life.

Corticosteroids — hormones produced by a part of the adrenal glands.

Diuretics — drugs capable of increasing the amount of urine passed.

Dysmenorrhea — pain with menstruation.

Endometrium — inner lining of the womb.

Estrogen — hormone produced by the ovaries.

Fallopian tubes — two tubes leading from the ovaries to the womb, along which the egg cells pass.

Geriatrics — care of the elderly.

Glaucoma — disease of the eye characterized by raised pressure in the eyeball.

Gynecology — study of the diseases of the woman.

Hormones — chemicals produced by glands, which pass in the bloodstream to exert an action at a distant site.

Hypothalamus — specialized part of the base of the brain concerned with control of metabolism.

Hysterectomy — surgical removal of the womb.

Implant — pellets of drugs inserted into the tissue.

Intermenstruum — part of the menstrual cycle not covered by the premenstruum or menstruation, usually days 5 to 24.

Intra-uterine device (IUD) — small contraceptive appliance inserted into the womb.

Menarche — first menstruation.

Menopause — last menstruation marking the end of the childbearing era.

Menstrual clock — the specialized portion of the hypo-thalamus responsible for the cyclical timing of menstruation.

Menstrual cycle — time from the first day of menstruation to the first day of the next menstruation.

Menstrual loss — bleeding at menstruation.

Menstruation — monthly bleeding from the vagina in women of childbearing age, caused by the disintegration of the lining of the womb.

Metabolism — building up and breaking down of chemicals in the body.

Migraine — severe form of headache.

Mittelschmerz — abdominal pain at the time of ovulation (middle pain).

Ovary — reproductive organ containing the egg cells.

Ovulation — release of the egg cell from the ovary.

Ovum — egg cell.

Paramenstruum — premenstruum and menstruation.

Pituitary — gland situated at the base of the brain and controlling many other glands.

Placebo — inert or inactive substance with no curative effect.

Postmenstruum — the days immediately after menstruation.

Post-natal — after childbirth.

Premenstruum — the days immediately prior to menstruation.

Pre-ovulatory — days before ovulation.

Progesterone — hormone produced by the ovary for the prepparation of the lining of the womb. Also a starting point for the production of numerous corticosteroids.

Progestogen — synthetic drugs used in contraceptives, once thought to be progesterone substitutes.

Prolactin — hormone produced by the pituitary gland.

Puerperium — after childbirth.

Spasmodic dysmenorrhea — spasms of pain occurring with menstruation.

Sterilization — operation to permanently prevent conception.

Synchrony — at the same time.

Syndrome — collection of symptoms which commonly occur together.

Testosterone — male hormone.

Therapy — treatment.

Uterus — womb.

Vagina — passage leading from the exterior of the body to the mouth of the womb

APPENDIX I

PMS: The Need for Legal Guidelines and Accurate Diagnosis

The seriousness of some aspects of premenstrual syndrome may result in the sufferer becoming involved in criminal proceedings. English courts have already accepted PMS as a mitigating factor if it is correctly diagnosed and confirmed by well-documented evidence of earlier episodes. In addition, there must be evidence of the patient's successful treatment with progesterone, which may need to be continued indefinitely to ensure that there is no future recurrence of criminal behavior.

PMS is a real hormone disorder and should not be overlooked as trivial, for this would be an injustice to the sufferer. On the other hand, to prevent abuse of the law by criminals, it is important that a clear legal definition of premenstrual syndrome (see Chapter 3) is accepted and thoroughly understood, that a defense formed on a plea of PMS is substantiated with fully documented dates of recurrent PMS-related incidents, and that a plea of PMS is used only in mitigation, as a contributing factor that is taken in consideration with other evidence. An overview of the subject was given in Chapter 14. In the following papers, the use of PMS arguments and the need for accurate diagnosis is covered in more detail. These papers were previously published in medical journals and are reproduced here for the serious reader and to help medical and legal researchers. Further and more recent work on the subject can be found in the list of the author's publications (pp. 199–201).

LEGAL IMPLICATIONS OF PMS

(Reprinted from **World Medicine,** April 1982)

[Note: The original style and spelling of the English publication has been retained in these following reprints.–*Ed.*]

A new responsibility has been placed on the medical profession as a result of the recent legal rulings recognising premenstrual syndrome (PMS) as a cause of diminished responsibility in two women charged with manslaughter. *It now becomes our duty to ensure that the plea of PMS will not be abused.* To do this will require that in every case the diagnosis of PMS is substantiated with incontrovertible evidence and that it will respond to treatment. Only the doctor can provide such evidence and ensure that the diagnosis is not abused.

Those few women who lose control of themselves for a day or two, month after month, need help and help is available. However, they must not be confused with the other 99.9 per cent of women who are well able to control their actions. PMS is not a universal defence, nor should it be allowed to become one. Medical evidence is required by the court and the doctor must become fully conversant with the recognition, diagnosis and treatment of the syndrome.

More than 30 years of research into PMS has produced a clear and precise definition: "the presence of *monthly recurrent* symptoms in the premenstruum or early menstruation with a *complete absence* of symptoms after menstruation." The words "monthly recurrent" and "complete absence" are essential in every correct diagnosis and the symptoms should have recurred in at least three consecutive menstrual cycles.

Furthermore, it must be borne in mind that at the PMS Clinic at University College Hospital, London, the diagnosis of PMS is confirmed in only half of the women claiming to have PMS. This is a similar figure to that noticed by Dr. Ronald Norris at the PMS Clinic in Boston, Mass.

The presence of "recurrent symptoms" implies that when a woman makes a plea of PMS at her first offence, that plea fails unless she can produce positive evidence of similar episodes of loss of control, confusion, amnesia or violence in the three previous cycles. Such evidence might be supplied by her employers, friends or family, or by searching through diaries, medical files, police records or prison documents.

The three cases of cyclical criminal charges in PMS reported in the *Lancet* in 1980(1) had been scrupulously researched. Indeed the woman charged with manslaughter had 30 previous convictions, occurring at cycles of 29.04 ± 1.47 days, and even while in prison had 26 episodes of bizarre behaviour including attempted strangling, drowning, attempted escape, slashing wrists, smashing windows and setting fire to her cell. These episodes, so meticulously documented by the prison officers on duty, occurred at intervals of 29.55 ± 1.45 days. The diagnosis did not rely on the woman's memory. Furthermore she was described as "pleasant and cooperative but at times she loses her senses and can be quite impulsive," which suggests that there was a complete absence of destructive symptoms after menstruation.

In contrast there is the case of a 22-year-old driver who made a successful plea at Burnham, Bucks, that PMS was the cause of her dangerous driving, as both crashes occurred within 48 hours of menstruation. She was not asked for additional evidence of any lapses of concentration in previous premenstruums, nor evidence of exemplary alertness in the postmenstruum. The occurrence of two crashes in the premenstruum could have been a mere coincidence.

In 1977 a 46-year-old part-time social worker faced a charge of shoplifting. In evidence she produced her diary showing the days of confusion each month, when she refused to leave the house, and she arranged her days at work accordingly. Her husband had recognised these cyclical occasions of confusion and described how she would return home from shopping with dog food, although they kept no animals, or a child ski outfit although their own children were now adult. Together with his wife, they had marked in the diary the days on which trouble might occur. All was well until a member of the staff caught the 'flu and the social worker agreed to alter her working days. The case was dismissed. She has since received progesterone treatment and been free from these lapses of concentration and confusion.

For a correct diagnosis of PMS the precise dates of menstruation and of the alleged crime are essential. A clerk in a travel agency was accused of stealing travellers cheques worth $1000 from her employer at some *unknown date* between August 1980 and April 1981. Her plea of PMS failed.

There are certain features which are characteristic of the offences committed by sufferers of PMS, which may be easily recognised.

1. The woman acts alone without an accomplice.
2. The offence is not premeditated, and usually comes as a surprise to those whom she was with shortly before the event.
3. The action is without apparent motive, such as setting fire to an unknown person's property.
4. There may be no attempt to escape detection. A woman randomly throwing a brick at a shop window may herself telephone the police and await her arrest.
5. The action may be a *cri de coeur*, as with the hoaxer who repeatedly makes emergency 999 calls. This is similar to a parasuicide.

Among the more frequent symptoms of PMS which may result in criminal charges are a sudden and momentary surge of uncontrollable emotions resulting in violence, confusion or amnesia, alcoholism, nymphomania and attention-seeking episodes which represent cries for help. These cover a full range of criminal offences such as actual violence, damage to property, theft and disorderly behaviour.

Sufferers of PMS characteristically have painfree menstruation. The shoplifter, who claimed her period pains were so severe that she was under the influence of pain-relieving drugs at the time of her offences, was suffering from spasmodic dysmenorrhoea and not from PMS. Incidentally, each of the three women reported in the *Lancet* was referred for a diagnosis of PMS by her father, who had noticed that his daughter's unpredictable behaviour occurred every four weeks. The three offenders had painfree menstruation and had not themselves associated this cyclical physiological event with their strange behaviour.

A full medical history will reveal many characteristic features, which confirm or refute the diagnosis. The onset of PMS, and the occasions of increased severity, always occur at times of hormonal upheaval, as at puberty, during or after taking the Pill, after amenorrhoea, pregnancy or sterilisation. These are the women who have side-effects on the Pill, and their pregnancy may be complicated by pre-eclampsia or postnatal depression. (2) During the premenstruum they have difficulty in tolerating long intervals without food (over five hours daytime or 13 hours overnight) and they become easily intoxicated by alcohol in the premenstruum.

A 32-year-old Essex housewife was accused of infanticide, having drowned her second daughter and then overdosed herself. She started menstruating in the intensive care unit and mention of PMS was noted in her previous medical records. She had developed migraine and hypertension on the Pill, for which she was admitted for observation to the London Hospital. Her first pregnancy was complicated by pre-eclampsia and after her second pregnancy she developed postnatal depression requiring a psychiatric domicilliary visit. The incident occurred about 5:30 p.m.; she had no food since her 8:30 a.m. breakfast. The court accepted the several diagnostic pointers of PMS and she was released on probation and treatment.

Among PMS women, increased libido is occasionally noticed in the premenstruum, a fact recorded by Israel back in 1938. All too often it is this nymphomanic urge in adolescents which is responsible for young girls running away from home, or custody, only to be found wandering in the park or following the boys. These girls can be helped, and their criminal career abruptly ended with hormone therapy.

Treatment with progesterone (not synthetic progestogen) is effective in well diagnosed cases of PMS, but not in menstrual distress, which is a term covering a multitude of disorders, including spasmodic dysmenorrhoea, endometriosis, hyperprolactinaemia, pelvic inflammatory disease, and symptoms of other diseases present through the cycle, but exacerbating during the paramenstruum, e.g., depression, neurosis, psychosis, migraine, arthritis, bronchitis.

Menstrual distress may be diagnosed by the use of the Moos Menstrual Distress Questionnaire (MMDQ) but this cannot be used for the diagnosis of PMS as it was not designed to reveal the recurrence of symptoms in the premenstruum or the absence in the postmenstruum, nor does it do so.

It is estimated that one in 10 of all menstruating women suffer from PMS severe enough to deserve treatment, but the proportion of sufferers charged with criminal offences is unknown. Some PMS women are needlessly detained and deserving of sympathy, and justice will not be done, or seen to be done, until the true sufferers are diagnosed and treated. PMS has been trivialized by the media and feminine interests will best be served by our ability to distinguish the few genuine sufferers from the many malingerers whose claims can never be substantiated.

REFERENCES
1. Dalton K. *Lancet* 1980;2:1070.
2. Dalton K. *Premenstrual Syndrome and Progesterone Therapy.* William Heinemann Medical Books, London, 1977.

THE IMPORTANCE OF DIAGNOSING PREMENSTRUAL SYNDROME

(Reprinted from **Health Visitor,** February 1982)

Introduction

In the 1950s, doctors were urged to look afresh at their chronic patients to ensure that they were not suffering from hidden depression which would respond to the newly discovered anti-depressants. Now, with our improved understanding of premenstrual syndrome (PMS), there is a similar need to take a new look at those chronic problem patients who are women in their menstruating years. We need to see whether they are victims of PMS who are suffering needlessly when they could be given the benefit of the highly successful treatment with natural progesterone.

Recently, premenstrual syndrome has been given legal recognition as a cause of diminished responsibility in murder, and as a mitigating factor in crimes of arson, assault, shoplifting and disorderly conduct. However, the law requires more than the mere statement that the woman was in her pre-menstruum at the time of her crime. Evidence must be produced to show that the symptoms recur regularly each month, and that treatment is likely to be successful and ensure that she will not repeat the offence.

Characteristics of PMS

Premenstrual syndrome is a disease of progesterone deficiency. The symptoms of PMS will therefore only occur in the second half of the menstrual cycle when adequate amounts of progesterone in the peripheral blood are required. After menstruation and until ovulation, progesterone is not present in the peripheral blood and so PMS symptoms will not occur. Therefore it follows that for the diagnosis of PMS it is essential to show that the timing of symptoms is limited to the premenstruum or early menstruation, with a complete absence of symptoms after menstruation. Diagnosis is best achieved by use of a menstrual chart on which the woman marks with an "M" the dates of menstruation (or with a "P" the dates of her period), and then uses other symbols for her symptoms, for example "X" for the days of quarrels, alcoholic bouts or asthma attacks, "T" for tiredness, "F" for forgetful days and "H" for headaches. Each woman can select symbols for her most troublesome symptoms. Charts are obtainable free from Cox-Continental Ltd, Brookside Avenue, Rustington, Sussex. Diagnosis rests on ensuring that there is a complete absence of symptoms during the postmenstruum. With a menstrual chart this diagnosis can be made at a glance, in fact even a ten-year-old child can recognize those charts which have no symbols for at least seven days after the "M"s.

Interviews with husbands and parents are invaluable, as those closest to the PMS sufferer will know best how she changes from the happy, charming individual which she is on most days into the lazy, irritable and unpredictable female she becomes as menstruation draws near.

Retrospective Diagnosis

In order to obtain a retrospective diagnosis it may be helpful to conduct searches elsewhere. Looking up the school register may reveal a monthly pattern of school truancy, as occurred in one teenager who was frightened to go to school on those days when his mother hit the bottle. Hospital records will show the precise dates of overdoses and self-mutilation attempts. The work register may be consulted to show cyclical absences, and police documents may display regular patterns of assault or drunk and disorderly behaviour. Even prison files may exhibit evidence of regular monthly episodes of bizarre behaviour occurring while in custody. All such information is valuable in building up positive evidence that the woman has symptoms at menstruation with normal behaviour at other times.

Other diagnostic pointers worth bearing in mind are the frequency with which the onset of PMS, and the occasions of increased severity, occur at times of upheaval of the menstrual hormones. These times include puberty, after pregnancy, during or after stopping the pill, after a spell of amenorrhea such as occurs in anorexia nervosa, and following sterilisation. Women with PMS usually have normal, pain-free and regular menstruation, and never experience the spasms of lower abdominal colicky pains so typical of spasmodic dysmenorrhoea.

Women with PMS are usually the ones who develop side effects on the pill, complaining that it causes headaches, depression or weight gain. They change their brand of pill and finally resort to some other contraceptive method. There is a high incidence of about nine women in every ten who develop PMS after certain complications associated with pregnancy. These include pre-eclampsia severe enough to require hospital admission in the antenatal period, or postnatal depression severe enough to need antidepressant treatment in the puerperium. There may also be a history of a threatened miscarriage in the early months with a successful outcome of pregnancy.

Body Chemistry

During the premenstruum, women with PMS experience a rise in glucose tolerance which results in food cravings and binges. The frequent weight gain and bloatedness in the premenstruum brings with it a desire to diet, so causing problems of intermittent feasting and famine. When PMS sufferers go too long without food, their blood glucose level reaches baseline and there is a compensating spurt of adrenalin to release glucose from the body's store. It is this sudden release of adrenalin which is responsible for many of the premenstrual symptoms such as panic attacks, explosive outbursts, uncontrollable aggression and migraine. After all, adrenalin is recognized as the hormone of fear, fight and flight. Careful enquiry will elicit the fact that most instances of baby battering and assault occur after a long food gap (five hours in the day or thirteen hours overnight). The mother who misses breakfast is most likely to be irritable at lunchtime, and the housewife who forgets her midday meal will be aggressive when her husband returns from work in the evening.

Alcohol tolerance varies over the menstrual cycle and those with PMS may find that during the premenstruum they are unable to tolerate their normal alcohol intake without signs of intoxication. The problem is increased by their urges to take alcohol at this time to overcome their premenstrual depression and lethargy. Thus during the premenstruum, at a time of lowered self-discipline, lowered self-control, alcohol urges and increased tendency to intoxication, is it any wonder that charges of drunk and disorderly occur with such frequency on the woman's charge sheets? Yet these same women may have no difficulty in totally abstaining from alcohol at other times of the menstrual cycle.

Conclusion

One in ten of all menstruating women are estimated to suffer from PMS severe enough to require treatment. Diagnosis is simple, but the responsibility of referring possible sufferers to their general practitioner frequently rests with health visitors, and they should not fail in this task.

Appendix II

PMS Clinics and
Support Groups
in the U.S.A. (1987)

This appendix is compiled from information received up to March 1, 1987, and is arranged in two parts. The first part comprises clinics with a medical director who accepts that premenstrual syndrome is a hormonal disease. Those marked with a "†" have attended a 2–4 day training course with Dr. Dalton.

The second part contains the names of PMS clinics and self-help groups with a non-medical director, whose approach may be psychological, nutritional, educational or herbal. Some are lay organizations which act as local referral agencies, others organize self-help groups, and most are able to put premenstrual syndrome sufferers in touch with physicians who understand progesterone therapy. Those marked with a "*" have a member of staff who has attended at least one lecture by Dr. Dalton. Both lists are organized alphabetically by state, and by zip code within each state.

Any such listing cannot remain up-to-date. To obtain more current information about individual doctors, clinics, or pharmacies compounding progesterone in specific areas, call the National PMS Society at 919-489-6577.

The inclusion of any group in these lists does *not* constitute a recommendation or endorsement of any kind by the author or the publishers, who cannot be held liable for any results from self-treatment, or treatment at any of the facilities listed in this book.

Part I

Alaska

† **The Health Care Center**   **(907) 562-7643**
200 W. 34th Ave., #364   W. Scott Kiester, D.O.
Anchorage, AK 99503   Jan Davis, R.N.
Physician-directed center for the diagnosis and treatment of PMS.

Arizona

† **333-Ob-Gyn Ltd. PMS Center**   **(602) 264-3267**
333 W. Thomas Rd., Ste. 211   Edward Sattenspieh, M.D.
Phoenix, AZ 85013   Donald E. Lee, M.D.
Doctors Sattenspieh and Lee have been trained and certified in the
treatment of PMS by Dr. Dalton.

† **PMS Institute**   **(602) 279-2233**
4541 N. 7th St.   Marshall Smith, M.D., Ph.D.
Phoenix, AZ 85014   Celia Halas, Ph.D.
A professional organization specializing in the evaluation and treatment of PMS. Also provides books, articles and tapes on PMS.

California

† **PMS Center**   **(213) 276-1151/1152**
9201 Sunset Blvd., Suite 906   Lloyd Byron Greig, M.D.
Los Angeles, CA 90069
Professional physician-directed clinic for the evaluation and treatment of PMS.

Connie Chein, M.D.   **(213) 274-8310**
9242 Olympic Blvd.   Dr. Connie Chein
Beverly Hills, CA 90212
Private medical practice specializing in the diagnosis and treatment
of PMS.

† **PMS Treatment Clinic**   **(818) 447-0679**
150 N. Santa Anita, #755   Richard Reitherman,M.D.
Arcadia, CA 91006   Holly Anderson
Offers treatment with natural progesterone therapy and provides
video presentations, books and tapes on PMS. Currently compiling
research data on SHBG test results.

† **PMS Medical Clinic of So. Cal.**   **(818) 798-9431/447-HELP**
2595 E. Washington Blvd.,Ste. 105   Thomas L. Riley, M.D.
Pasadena, CA 91107   Rayne Dawson, P.A.-C.
Offers counseling, nutritional and vitamin therapy, exercise programs, and natural progesterone therapy.

Charter Oak Hospital PMS Clinic   **(818) 966-1632**
1161 E. Covina Blvd.   Perry Maloff, M.D.
Covina, CA 91724   Lynn Foerster, Ph.D.
Provides education, evaluation, and a multi-disciplinary approach to
the treatment of PMS.

San Diego PMS Clinic   **(619) 297-3311**
591 Camino de la Reina, Suite 533   Dr. Lori Futterman
San Diego, CA 92108   Dr. M. E. Ted Quigley
Professional practice which diagnoses, treats, researches and educates
about PMS.

Special Problems in Gynecology   **(800) CAL-4-PMS**
720 N. Tustin Ave., #203   Stanley Lubell, M.D.
Santa Ana, CA 92705   Bonnie Lawrence
Provides diagnosis and treatment using hormone therapy, diet and
nutrition, biofeedback and exercise. Also provides charting diaries
and books on PMS.

Women's Lifecare Medical Centers, Inc.   **(714) 974-3472**
500 S. Anaheim Hills Rd., Ste. 200   Harinder Grewal, M.D.
Anaheim Hills, CA 92807   Ria Gagnon
Provides hormonal, biochemical, nutritional and psychosocial evaluations and treatments of PMS, postpartum depression and post-
hysterectomy syndrome.

Burlingame PMS Clinic   **(415) 697-7211**
1828 El Camino Real, Ste. 504   William Rosenzweig, M.D.
Burlingame, CA 94010   Corinne Carrigan
Professional physician-directed organization specializing in individualized dietary and vitamin supplementation programs. Uses natural
progesterone therapy if needed.

Colorado

PMS Treatment Center   **(303) 869-1504/83-WOMEN**
Women's Hospital at AMI St. Lukes   William E. Fuller, M.D.
601 E. 19th Avenue   Judith Ensign, M.S., R.N., C.F.N.P.
Denver, CO 80203
Professional, physician-directed organization which diagnoses and
treats PMS. Also provides information, education, and support groups
for the community.

PMS Clinic   **(303) 440-7100**
2760 29th St., Ste. 205   Jed Shapiro, M.D.
Boulder, CO 80301   Stephanie Bender, M.A.
Professional, physician-supervised organization specializing in the education and evaluation of PMS. Individual and family counseling is also available.

Florida

The Florida PMS Clinics, Inc.   **(305) 271-8808**
11400 N. Kendall Dr., Ste. 212   Dr. E. Gail Brown
Miami, FL 33176   Jeannette Brown, R.N., M.A.
A network of health professionals who provide support groups and individualized assessment and management of PMS.

Georgia

† **The Douglass Center**   **(404) 953-0710**
2470 Windy Hill Road, Ste. 440   William C. Douglass, M.D.
Marietta, GA 30067   Carol Carter
Provides progesterone therapy, individual nutrition plans and vitamin supplementation, and PMS literature. Dr. Douglass maintains regular contact with Dr. Dalton.

Hawaii

PMS Hawaii   **(808) 538-7164/523-0027**
1380 Lusitania St.   H. Lorrin Lau, M.D.
Honolulu, HI 96813   Amy Voshall
PMS Hawaii offers lectures and support sessions for PMS sufferers. Dr. Lau's office treats menstrual problems and is forming a multi-disciplinary team to research PMS.

Kansas

† **Glenn O. Bair, M.D.**   **(913) 267-3025/5689**
2300 West 29th St., Ste. 123   Glenn O. Bair, M.D.
Topeka, KS 66611   Charlotte Elder, R.N.
Private practice specializing in the diagnosis and treatment of PMS according to the precepts of Dr. Dalton.

† **U. of Kansas School of Medicine, Wichita**   **(316) 261-2622**
Internal Medicine Clinic   Robert T. Manning, M.D.
1010 N. Kansas
Wichita, KS 67214
Provides diagnostic evaluation and therapeutic planning for PMS sufferers.

Maryland

PMS Treatment Center   (301) 330-2666/984-9791
5918 Hubbard   Dr. Bruce A. Kehr, M.D.
Rockville, MD 20852   Crystal Marcus, L.C.S.W.
Professional organization which evaluates women with PMS and provides a comprehensive individualized treatment program.

PMS Treatment Center   (301) 977-4114
507 N. Frederick Ave.   Jeffrey Levitt, M.D.
Gaithersburg, MD 20877   Stephen R. Goldburg, M.D.
Provides PMS diagnosis and treatment, including prostaglandin inhibitors and natural progesterone.

Massachusetts

Manjul Shukla, M.D.   (617) 752-1702
7 Bellevue St.   Dr. Manjul Shukla
Worcester, MA 01609
Private practice specializing in diagnosis and treatment of PMS.

† **Michelle Harrison, M.D.**   (617) 491-5800
763 Massachusetts Ave.   Dr. Michelle Harrison
Cambridge, MA 02139
Specializes in the diagnosis and treatment of PMS and particularly in separating PMS from psychiatric illness.

Minnesota

PMS Discovery, Support & Training Center   (612) 472-5311
5023 Edgewater Dr.   M. Siefert, M. D.
Mound, MN 55364   Joy Bennet
Professional organization specializing in support groups, workshops, individual evaluations, and physician referral.

Wellness Center of Minnesota   (507) 345-7898
Good Counsel   Dr. William D. Manahan, M.D.
Mankato, MN 56001   Carl Lofy, S.T.D.; Linda Hachfeld, R.D.
Offers counseling and nutrition planning which emphasizes wellness of the whole person.

Missouri

† **PMS Center of St. Louis**   (314) 727-3087
950 Francis Pl.   John B. Bennett, M.D.
Clayton, MO 63105
Dr. Bennett was trained by Dr. Dalton and follows her treatment methods.

† **PMS Program Center**   **(314) 997-3333**
443 N. New Ballas Road   Godofredo Herzog, M.D.
Suite 240   Patricia C. Coughlin, R.N., Ph.D.
St. Louis, MO 63141   Catherine L. Fox
Program screens, diagnoses and treats PMS and offers education, nutritional guidance and self-help groups.

† **PMS Carecenter**   **(816) 444-4232/4322**
Rockhill Medical Building, Ste. 502   Mary C. Cortner, M.D.
6700 Troost Ave.   Joan Wood
Kansas City, MO 64131
Physician-directed professional organization providing detailed evaluation and treatment of PMS. The Center's staff is trained and approved by Dr. Dalton.

New York

Manhattan PMS Center   **(212) 861-4580**
1520 York Ave., Ste. 26B   Sondra L. Carter, M.D.
New York, NY 10028   Lynn A. Greenfield, R.N.
Professional organization providing evaluation and treatment of PMS, and support groups for PMS sufferers and their families.

North Carolina

† **Duke Univ. Medical Center PMS Clinic**   **(919) 684-5322**
Box 3263 Duke University Medical Center   John Steege, M.D.
Durham, NC 27710   Sharon Rupp
Provides a multi-disciplinary evaluation approach by a gynecologist, psychologist and nurse practioner.

Ohio

Women's Center   **(513) 241-9506/621-1698**
173 East McMillan St.   Martin Haskell, M.D.
Cincinnati, OH 45219   Claudia Dehner, O.G.N.P.
Diagnoses and treats PMS from a natural, psychological, and medical perspective. Offers natural progesterone therapy and a support group.

Women's Med Plus Center of Dayton   **(513) 293-3917**
1401 E. Stroop Rd., Ste. 6   Martin Haskell, M.D.
Dayton, OH 45429   Adele Dean R.N.C.; Diane Wissman, R.N.
Offers physician-directed diagnosis and treatment including diet, exercise, relaxation techniques, counseling and natural progesterone therapy.

Oregon

PMS Treatment Center   **(503) 255-0918**
10373 N.E. Hancock   Phil Alberts, M.D., F.A.C.O.G.
P.O. Box 20998   Suzanne L. Alberts, R.N.C.
Portland, OR 97220-0998
Provides national referral service in addition to a local multi-disciplinary diagnostic, treatment and education program.

Pennsylvania

Matrix PMS Clinic   **(412) 782-2992/4700**
135 Freeport Road   Christiane M. F. Siewers, M.D.
Pittsburgh, PA 15215   Mary Kay Lewis
Provides comprehensive treatment, including diet, exercise, nutrition, natural progesterone and minidose progesterone therapy, and psychotherapy or counseling if desired.

U. of Pennsylvania PMS Program   **(215) 662-3329**
Department of Ob./Gyn.   Steven J. Sondheimer, M.D.
Hospital of the U. of Pennsylvania   Ellen W. Freeman, Ph.D.
3400 Spruce St.
Philadelphia, PA 19104
Non-profit program evaluating and treating PMS in a research context focused on treatment effectiveness and the endocrine effects in PMS. Progesterone treatment is free to study participants.

Marvin R. Hyett, M.D.   **(215) 928-4800**
1100 Walnut St.   Dr. Marvin R. Hyett
Philadelphia, PA 19107
Private practice specializing in diagnosis and treatment of PMS, using multiple approaches including progesterone therapy. Also has offices in Northfield, NJ, and Cherry Hill, NJ.

Tennessee

Vanderbilt University PMS Program   **(615) 322-6573**
Center for Fertility & Reproductive Research
Vanderbilt U. Medical Center North   Joel Hargrove, M.D.
Room D-3223, Nashville, TN 37232
Physician-directed clinic for evaluation and treatment of PMS.

Texas

PMS Center of Irving Texas   (214) 579-0551
1430 MacArthur, Ste. 103   Frank Knopp, M.D.
Irving, TX 75061
Physician-directed center for PMS diagnosis and treatment, including
progesterone therapy.

Albert M. Kincheloe, D.O.   (817) 265-9928
2625 Matlock, #103   Dr. Albert M. Kincheloe
Arlington, TX 76015   Cheryl Kincheloe
Private practice providing PMS treatment with natural progesterone,
nutrition, diet and exercise.

† **PMS Program**   (713) 799-8047/8494
Women's Hospital of Texas   Louise A. Bednar Terril, M.D.
7600 Fannin   Cindy Dear, R.N., M.S.
Houston, TX 77054   Jackie Lancaster, R.N. A.D.N.
Evaluates, diagnoses, and treats PMS. The program's physician and
director were trained by Dr. Dalton.

Utah

Utah PMS Center at the Western Institute   (801) 584-2105
501 Chipeta Way   Richard Shanteau, M.D.
Salt Lake City, UT 84108   Kathie Smith, R.N.
Provides diagnosis, medical treatment, education and support for
women suffering from PMS and related problems.

Wisconsin

Eau Claire Clinic, Ltd.   (715) 834-3171
2103 Heights Dr., Box 264   Albert A. Lorenz, M.D.
Eau Claire, WI 54702   Sharon A. Heinz, M.S.E.
Private psychiatric clinic providing assessment, education, and physician-directed treatment (including nutrition, life style changes, and
progesterone therapy).

Part II

Alaska

* **PMS Support of Ketchikan**   (907) 225-5827/6425
815 Brown Deer Rd.   Patricia Francis
Ketchikan, AK 99901   Candi Kock
Offers information, support, and medical referral to physicians who
treat PMS according to Dr. Dalton's treatment plan.

California

* **Family Resource Center**   (213) 476-8561, ext. 209
Stephen S. Wise Temple   Marilyn Brown, Director
15500 Stephen S. Wise Dr.   Norma Freeman, M.F.C.C.
Los Angeles, CA 90077
Provides education and support for PMS sufferers and their families.
Dr. Dalton is a consultant to the program.

St. Joseph's Hospital Community Education   (714) 771-8040
1100 W. Stewart Dr.   Mecca Carpenter, Ph.D.
Orange, CA 92668
Offers local physician referrals and information through literature and
videotapes on PMS and women's health issues.

* **PMS Action, Inc.**   (714) 786-8775
P.O. Box 16292   Virginia Cassara
Irvine, CA 92713   Linda Jones
National, non-profit organization providing information and referrals
to physicians using natural progesterone therapy.

Feminine Resources for PMS   (415) 937-4342
P.O. Box 1762   Roseann Parker
Lafayette, CA 94549
Self-help oriented organization which provides physician referrals,
group support classes and one-night workshops.

Health Options/Resources for PMS   (408) 476-4956
P.O. Box 1917   Marilyn Seach Koll
Aptos, CA 95001
Provides extensive referrals to physicians and health care profes-
sionals, self-help and education materials, seminars and lectures.

PMS Network, Inc.   **(916) 969-8237**
P.O. Box 162792   Gail Lesh, M.P.H.
Sacramento, CA 95816   Lesley Schroeder, M.D.
Provides educational information about PMS, workshops, support groups and physician referrals in the Sacramento Valley.

PMS Relief   **(916) 823-9930**
7955 Bullard Dr.   Gillian Ford
Newcastle, CA 95658
Provides education and counseling in association with several physicians who treat according to Dr. Dalton's approach.

Colorado

PMS Clinic of Western Colorado   **(303) 245-6321**
Centennial Plaza, Suite 30   Nancy T. Wilson, M.A.
2721 N. 12th Street   Carolynn S. Nelson, M.A., N.C.C.
Grand Junction, CO 81506
Provides treatment for PMS sufferers, with a strong emphasis on psychological aspects. Holds meetings and seminars for sufferers and their families.

Connecticut

PMS Treatment Center of Hartford   **(203) 688-0393**
34 Maple Ave.   JoAnn Mizell, R.N.
Windsor, CT 06095
Specializes in the treatment of PMS, and post-partum and menopausal distress. Offers support groups and referrals.

Florida

Gainsville Women's Health Center   **(904) 377-5055**
720 N.W. 23rd Ave.   Judith Whitley, A.R.N.P.
Gainesville, FL 32606
Non-profit women's clinic which initiates treatment of PMS with diet, vitamins, counseling and exercise. Provides physician referrals for further treatment.

Illinois

* **Fox Valley PMS Center**   **(312) 897-5616**
648 N. Randall Rd.   William H. Woodruff, M.D.
Aurora, IL 60506   Peg Sechrest, R.N.C., Judy Barr, C.S.T.
Evaluates and treats PMS with diet, exercise, vitamins, and progesterone. Also offers a PMS support group.

Indiana

Westside Guidance PMS Program   (317) 241-7065
Indianapolis PMS Support Group
805 Beachway Dr., #110   Linda Cameron
Westlake Medical Building   Norma Kistner, R.N., B.S.N.
Indianapolis, IN 46224
Private, out-patient psychiatric clinic provides evaluation and treat-
ment through the services of health professionals. Natural proges-
terone therapy is used in severe cases. The Indianapolis PMS Support
Group is an affiliated non-profit organization providing literature and
charting instructions on PMS.

The Wellness Center   (219) 736-1025/947-2088
8080 Utah St.   Sharon J. Wendt, Ph.D.
Merrillville, IN 46410   Kathie Smith, R.N.
Provides consultation, examinations and diagnosis. Also offers nutritional management with diet and vitamin therapy, hormone therapy,
support groups, and PMS seminars.

PMS Community Awareness   (812) 372-5340
1914 Chandler Lane   Laurie Woodall
Columbus, IN 47203
Non-professional phone counseling service.

Iowa

North Iowa Women's Center   (515) 421-5491
910 N. Eisenhower   Maxine Brinkman, B.S.N.
Mason City, IA 50401   Jeannie Bitker, B.S.N.
Provides assessment and education, including charting instructions,
diet therapy, counseling, and physician referrals.

Kansas

Premenstrual Support Group   (316) 268-6767/5993
St. Francis Regional Medical Center   Alberta McGreevy, R.N.
929 N. St. Francis   Helen Ven John, R.N.
Wichita, KS 67214
Support group for PMS sufferers; also provides physician referrals.

Massachusetts

Women's Health and Nutrition Center   **(413) 549-6808**
320 N. Pleasant St., P.O. Box 628   JoAnn Mizell, R.N.
Amherst, MA 01004
Specializes in the treatment of PMS, post-partum and menopausal distress. Offers support groups and physician referrals.

* **Northshore Women's Care**   **(617) 942-0743**
511 Pearl St.   Laurea Nugent, R.N.C.
Reading, MA 01867   Dr. Richard McDowell
Ms. Nugent is an OB/GYN nurse practitioner who specializes in work with PMS patients and has attended Dr. Dalton's workshops.

Michigan

PMS Services, Inc.   **(616) 327-2134**
8135 Cox's Dr.   Susan Stewart
Portage, MI 49002
Screens and counsels women referred by physicians. Offers evaluations, pattern charts, education, diet, exercise and vitamins. Referrals to physicians for progesterone therapy.

Minnesota

PMS Clinic of Minneapolis, Inc.   **(612) 830-0990**
Edina Professional Building #200   Jane A. Trimble, R.N., M.S.
7250 France Ave. S.
Minneapolis, MN 55435
Provides comprehensive evaluation, treatment, support and education services for women with PMS.

Montana

Planned Parenthood of Billings: PMS Program   **(406) 248-3636**
721 N. 29th St.   Clayton McCracken, M.D.
Billings, MT 59101   Jean Omelchuck
Provides physician referrals throughout the state as well as PMS assessment, treatment, education, support and literature.

New Jersey

James Street Chiropractic Center   (201) 285-0888
12 James St.   Dr. Michael W. Gervis
Morristown, NJ 07960
Provides a natural approach to PMS relief including gentle spinal
manipulation, physcial therapy, diet and exercise.

North Carolina

National PMS Society   (919) 489-6577
1106 W. Corwallis Rd., Office 105   Kitty Johnson
Durham, NC 27706
Provides support, information and advocacy for PMS sufferers. Also
offers referral to doctors, clinics, support groups and pharmacists
compounding natural progesterone.

North Dakota

PMS Support League   (701) 775-0457
221 S. Fourth St.   Sue Yarbro
Grand Forks, ND 58201   Joyce Ring
Provides referrals to local physicians. Offers self-help manual, support
groups for PMS sufferers and families, lectures, seminars and other
educational resources.

Ohio

Guidance Center of Ashland   (419) 289-2522
738 Claremont Ave.   Roger D. Osborn, Ph.D.
Ashland, OH 44805   N. Ruth Mistie, W.S.W.
Provides PMS education and referral.

Oregon

Biological Research Collegium   (503) 342-3004
3977 Dillard Rd.   Raymond Peat, Ph.D.
Eugene, OR 97405   Leslie Scott
Provides non-medical support, classes based on Dr. Dalton's work,
and physician referrals for natural progesterone treatment.

Tennessee
PMS Newsletter and Support   **(615) 896-3025**
P.O. Box 2894   Pam Hoard, C.S.A.C.
Murfreesboro, TN 37133
Networks nationally to provide referrals for PMS treatment and re-
sources for progesterone therapy. Offers support, education, and a
non-profit PMS newsletter.

Texas

* **PMS Counseling and Education**   **(512) 372-3179**
P.O. Box 1735   Gail Post, R.N., M.S.
Seguin, TX 78155
Provides individual counseling, seminars and presentations for PMS
patients, and physician referral.

Virginia

* **WomensCare Corporation**   **(703) 255-2125**
8998 Kildownet Court   Patty Cannon
Vienna, VA 22180
Offers consultation in the establishment of hospital-based comprehensive PMS clinics.

Washington

Elspeth Wallace, R.N.   **(206) 363-6505**
3504 N.E. 162nd Ave.   Elspeth Wallace
Seattle, WA 98155
Provides education, charting instructions, evaluation and management of symptoms, counseling, classes, support activities and physician referrals.

PMS Support Group of Othello   **(509) 488-3139**
475 Fircrest   Teresa Potter
Othello, WA 99344
Offers monthly support group, monthly meetings with guest speakers,
and local pharmacy and physician referrals.

Wisconsin
PMS Program   **(414) 258-2600**
Milwaukee Psychiatric Hospital   Peg Miota, B.S.N.
1220 Dewey Ave.   Mary Yahle, R.N., C.S.
Wauwatosa, WI 53213
Promotes awareness of women's health and encourages natural ther-
apy techniques.

PMS Access   **(800) 222-4PMS/in WI (608) 833-4PMS**
P.O. Box 9326   Marla Ahlgrimm, R.Ph.
Madison, WI 53715
National clearinghouse for PMS information. Provides toll-free infor-
mation line, bi-monthly newsletter, referrals to physicians and support
groups, and a wide selection of educational materials.

Family Life Education PMS Program   **(414) 433-3584**
Bellin Hospital   Judy Medress, B.S.
744 South Webster Ave.
P. O. Box 1700
Green Bay, WI 54301
Provides education and support for PMS sufferers and their families.
Staff members were trained by PMS Action.

PMS Support Group   **(608) 784-5366/788-1308**
W5655 Hwy. 33, #38   Ann Hudson
La Crosse, WI 54601
Self-help group for PMS sufferers.

Fox Valley Reproductive Health Care   **(414) 731-9534**
3800 N. Gillet   Maggie Cage
Appleton, WI 54912   Debbie Sage
Offers screening, education, advocacy and support, and physician
referrals to PMS sufferers.

Index